D0392091

THE SPARK

Also by Dr. Glenn A. Gaesser

Big Fat Lies: The Truth About Your Weight and Your Health

Also by Karla Dougherty

True-Life Ghost Stories

(with Richard C. Senelick, M.D.)

Beyond Please and Thank You: The Disability Sensitivity Handbook for Families, Co-Workers, and Friends
The Spinal Cord Injury Handbook for Patients and Their Families
Living with Stroke: A Guide for Families (with Richard C. Senelick, M.D., and Peter W. Ross, M.D.)

(with Stephen J. Rosenberg, M.D.)

The Pocket Idiot's Guide to First Aid

(with James M. Rippe, M.D.)

The Polar Fat-Free and Fit Forever Program
The Rockport Walking Program (with James M. Rippe, M.D., and Ann Ward, Ph.D.)

THE SPARK

A Revolutionary New Plan to Get Fit
and Lose Weight 10 Minutes at a Time

Dr. Glenn A. Gaesser and Karla Dougherty

RODALE

Notice

This book is intended as a reference volume only, not as a medical manual. The information given here is designed to help you make informed decisions about your health. It is not intended as a substitute for any treatment that may have been prescribed by your doctor. If you suspect that you have a medical problem, we urge you to seek competent medical help. As with any exercise program, check with your doctor before you begin.

Mention of specific companies, organizations, or authorities in this book does not imply endorsement by the publisher, nor does mention of specific companies, organizations, or authorities in the book imply that they endorse the book.

A previous version of this book was published by Simon & Schuster.

Copyright © 2001 by Glenn A. Gaesser, Ph.D., and Karla Dougherty
Illustrations copyright © 2001 by Jackie Aher

All rights reserved. No part of this publication may be reproduced or transmitted in any form or by any means, electronic or mechanical, including photocopying, recording, or any other information storage and retrieval system, without the written permission of the publisher.

Printed in the United States of America
Rodale Inc. makes every effort to use acid-free ∞, recycled paper ♻.

Designed by Stratford Publishing Services, Inc.

Library of Congress Cataloging-in-Publication Data

Gaesser, Glenn A. (Glenn Alan)
    The spark : a revolutionary new plan to get fit and lose weight 10 minutes at a time / Glenn A. Gaesser and Karla Dougherty.
        p.   cm.
    Originally published by Simon & Schuster with subtitle: the revolutionary 3-week fitness plan that changes everything you know about exercise, weight control, and health.
    Includes indexes.
    ISBN 1–57954–511–4   hardcover
    1. Exercise.   2. Physical fitness.   3. Nutrition.   4. Health.   I. Dougherty, Karla.
II. Title.
RA781 .G334   2001b
613.7—dc21   2001019874

2 4 6 8 10 9 7 5 3   hardcover

Visit us on the Web at www.rodalestore.com, or call us toll-free at (800) 848-4735.

RODALE

WE **INSPIRE** AND **ENABLE** PEOPLE TO IMPROVE
THEIR LIVES AND THE WORLD AROUND THEM

DR. GLENN A. GAESSER
*To the Sparks of my life—Mike, Lindsay, and Brandon;
and the flame—Patricia*

KARLA DOUGHERTY
To my husband, D.J., my partner forever on the ride of my life

CONTENTS

Acknowledgments 9

Before You Spark . . . 13

Chapter 1: What Is the Spark? 15

Chapter 2: Why the Spark? 32

Chapter 3: Making the Spark Work for You:
A Series of Self-Tests 62

Chapter 4: The Basic Spark Exercise Plan 98

Chapter 5: The Basic Spark Food Plan 125

Chapter 6: Week One: Embers 149

Chapter 7: Week Two: Kindling 161

Chapter 8: Week Three: The Fire and Beyond—
Finessing the Spark 180

Appendix A: A Week of Spark Sample Exercise
and Food Menus 207

Contents

Appendix B: Spark Recipes   225

Appendix C: Three-Week Spark Exercise and Fiber Log   381

                Index   384

                Recipe Index   393

                Conversion Chart   400

ACKNOWLEDGMENTS

As with any endeavor, this book is more than the two of us. If we had not had the help and support of the following people, *The Spark* would have never existed. To them we give thanks:

The forty members of the initial Spark Study 2000. Without their commitment and faith, there would have been no proof to back up our words;

Our literary agents, Richard Parks and Lynn Seligman. They were the matches that ignited the first Spark;

Sydny Miner, our editor at Simon & Schuster, who not only believed in this book so much that she wanted to publish it, but who shares our vision of what the Spark is;

Jackie Aher, whose illustrations grace the pages of this book;

Joelle Delbourgo, who was the first person who said, "Go for it!"

In addition, Dr. Gaesser would like to thank his colleagues and students, past and present, who have contributed so much to his understanding of the link among exercise, diet, and health. A special thanks to Dr. Eugene Barrett, at the University of Virginia, without whose support and generosity the Spark Study 2000 would not have been possible; and to Linda Jahn, one of the most genuine and dedicated persons with whom he has ever had the pleasure to work. Also, a debt

Acknowledgments

of gratitude to Karin Kratina, for her wonderful work on hunger, nutrition, and people's relationships with food.

Karla Dougherty will always feel deep gratitude to her cousins Gail McGovern and "little Stevie" Rosenberg, who first put the idea of the Boston–New York AIDS Ride into her head; Christene and Arthur Mann, who redefined the meaning of good friends and neighbors; Dr. Rose Oosting, who offered wisdom and kindness when she needed it most; Fran Pelzman Liscio, who has always been a source of profound inspiration; Jennifer Wasky, who helped her get fit even when it was the last thing she wanted to do; and to all her friends who were there for her, offering encouragement even as they wondered who she'd become. And, finally, a special thanks to all the people she'd met on every Ride she'd ever done and to all the everyday heroes who courageously ride out their lives from day to day.

"From a small spark,
Great flame has risen."
—DANTE

BEFORE YOU SPARK . . .

In these pages you will discover not only new truths about exercise and diet, fitness and weight, but a new approach.

Your guide will be Dr. Glenn Gaesser, the scientist behind the groundbreaking Spark Study 2000 at the University of Virginia, a research project that helped bring its forty participants to a new level of health and vitality.

Coauthor Karla Dougherty, at fifty, found her Spark quite by accident and recounts her fight from the fitness trenches in passages entitled *K's Spark*.

Read this book, listen to its message, and you will find your own Spark.

CHAPTER 1

What Is the Spark?

On May 10, at 1:12 P.M., Jon Krakauer, one of the survivors of the ill-fated 1996 Mount Everest expedition, made it to the top: 29,028 feet above sea level, the highest point in the world and the intense, shining focus of the past two months. He stayed at the summit, one foot in China, one in Nepal, for approximately 10 minutes.

It's an old cliché that academics in ivory towers are not in touch with everyday folks. You wouldn't necessarily put exercise physiologists in that group. After all, we deal with activity: we're out there on the tracks, in the parks, at the gym.

You'd be wrong. We might run up those ivory towers two steps at a time, but we still inhabit them.

This revelation came to me in 1999, a year after I had convened with my fellow academics of the American College of Sports Medicine to establish the new fitness guidelines for maximum health and longevity.

It was then, in a series of conference calls, e-mails, faxes, and meetings, that we proudly and concisely compiled research, statistics, and data that had accumulated over the past eight years. Our recommendations?

Perform intense aerobic workouts, 20 to 60 minutes at a time, 3 to 5 times a week, combined with 2 to 3 times a week of both strength-training and flexibility exercises.

You've heard this all before. These guidelines have formed the basis of countless magazine articles, books, gymnastics programs, "join this gym" inducements, even infomercials. So what's the problem?

Well, let's put these recommendations another way:

Intense, sweat-inducing exercise.

Twenty minutes to a full hour.

Three to five days a week.

Spend your days off lifting weights.

And find an hour somewhere in there to stretch.

Now, there definitely are individuals out there who would—and who have—embraced these guidelines. There are people who exercise at least three days a week at an intensity that would make ice burn. I'm one of them; it's my business and my passion. But it's certainly not a way of life for most Americans.

It occurred to me after that day in 1999 that our fitness guidelines were completely unrealistic. That our "ivory tower" mentality encouraged people to start an exercise program over and over again, only to fail and become even more sedentary than before. That our unrealistic expectations motivated people to join health clubs and never set foot in the places after the first three months.

In other words, these guidelines, constructed by myself and my colleagues with the utmost commitment to the health of all Americans, have actually contributed to making Americans *five to ten pounds heavier* than they were a generation ago!

But there's more. Not only did we ask Americans to carve out a good portion of their harried week, we also asked them to be patient. All the studies we used to compose our fitness guidelines of course showed significant improvement—*but only after following an exercise regimen for three months or longer.*

Finally, the third and last revelation hit me: Each study, detailed and meticulous as it was, concentrated on only one or two elements of fitness at a time. There were studies that concentrated on cardiovascular health. Aerobic capacity. Strength training. Flexibility and joint range of motion. Metabolic fitness and weight loss. But there was no one study that combined all these different aspects of fitness to see what the results might be.

The scientist in me began to hypothesize. I kept going back to the first page of the printed guidelines where, in parentheses, almost as an afterthought, we stated that a daily workout of at least half an hour could be broken up into 10-minute segments if necessary throughout the day. "What ifs" began to occupy my waking hours. What if a standard exercise program was made even shorter? What if you added strength training and flexibility into the 10-minute equation? What if you never had to do any exercise for more than 10 minutes at a time? Would you still get positive results—especially in older, more sedentary individuals? And what if you combined these 10-minute bouts of exercise or *Sparks* with a concrete diet plan? Would you still lose weight?

And the biggest question of all: How long would it take to see results?

Enter the three-week Spark study at the University of Virginia.

(continued on page 20)

K's Spark

It was the ruins at Mesa Verde that got me. These ancient Indian dwellings, thousands of years old, were once inhabited by a tribe that carved out lives from dozens of rocky cliffs. Their stone-and-clay homes had sheltered a people who were active from morning until night: farming, harvesting, cooking, praying. Exercise with a purpose: survival.

But that hot summer morning, when my husband, D.J., and I headed for their hills, we weren't thinking about ancient civilizations, and we certainly weren't thinking about exercising. We were thinking about fun. We were on our first vacation in years and we felt giddy with freedom. We'd heard that Mesa Verde, in southwest Colorado, was an awesome site.

The only problem with Mesa Verde is that if you want to see the clay buildings, you have to go on your own body power.

That means climbing hills. Steep hills. But there we were, armed with water and sunscreen, ready for adventure in the hot Rocky Mountain sun.

I was wearing comfortable hiking shoes and shorts. Although my outfit showed every ounce of the forty pounds I'd gained over the past few years, I didn't see it. To me, I was the fairly slim person I'd been in my twenties.

This illusion stuck with me all the way down the first slope. It was easy. Nothing to it but a wayward rock or two. But by the time we hiked the uphill path to the first ruin, I was out of breath and sweating.

My heart hadn't stopped pounding in my ears, but I chose to ignore it. I distracted myself by imagining the Indians stoking a fire in the earth, murmuring softly in their ancient tongue, waking to the sharp slats of sun coming through slits in their hut's clay wall.

After about a half hour, we'd seen everything there was to see. It was time to move on. **To walk back up the cliff.**

No problem, I told myself. My heart had stopped pounding; my breath seemed less ragged. I began to climb. One step. Two. Maybe three or four. I lost count. I was too busy trying to breathe. The edge of the cliff seemed distant, surrounded by a halo of light. The top! I'd never make it.

I continued to climb—and stopped every few feet. Climb. Stop. Gasp. Climb. Stop. Gasp. D.J. had already gone up to the crest. I couldn't even see him anymore. I drank my water. Climb. Stop. Gasp.

I wasn't alone. There was a group of women who kept up the same pace, maybe a few years older than I from the looks of them. (To be honest, when I caught enough breath to glance at them, they looked *much* older and, of course, *much, much* heavier than I.)

We complained and commiserated with one another as we did the "Mesa Verde Walk." Climb. Stop. Gasp. We made jokes about how the Anasazis must have climbed up these hills. "Hope they hadn't forgotten anything." "So this is why they disappeared." I could barely laugh, let alone stand. Somehow, probably from the sheer terror of embarrassment that a park ranger might have to carry me up, I got to the top of the cliff. I fell onto a nearby bench. I sat and breathed, hard; the air felt like rocks. I waved good-bye to my new friends—who, oddly, seemed to be recovering more easily than I (*especially* for their age and weight!).

Five, then ten minutes. I sat, still breathing hard. I pretended I wasn't having as bad a time adjusting as I really was, so D.J. wouldn't be too worried. But I was scared. I was afraid that I was having a heart attack—at forty-eight.

I almost wanted to die. I would rather die, I thought, than face this particular fear: that I had let myself go. That I was fat. That I was in worse shape than people who were my mother's age. That I had become that person whom I'd never wanted to be, heavy, unfit, old before my time. How did this happen?

In many ways, my studies on the Spark were a natural progression, from my active childhood growing up in the '60s to my position as cochair on the American College of Sports Medicine fitness guidelines committee. I can't remember a time when I wasn't moving, running, sprinting, jumping. I never sat still. If there was a football game or a baseball game, or even an hour to throw around a few balls, I was there. Being active was a way of life. I just didn't know that a sedentary lifestyle was an option.

In high school, I discovered that I was good at running, that I had a high aerobic capacity. I ran competitively and won a couple of awards. Even today, if I don't get my run in on a daily basis, I'm uncomfortable. I miss the physical, emotional, and spiritual "high."

It was this passion for movement that led me to study exercise physiology at Berkeley, where I studied peak performance in athletes. I loved my work and enjoyed publication in many journals and a professorship at the University of Virginia.

But something happened along the way. Athletes stopped being a challenge. I began to wonder why I was spending so much time and effort on such a small percentage of the population. My interest began to shift to the general public, in particular to the vast number of people who really needed solid, helpful information on good health and fitness.

With funding from the American Heart Association, I began my research on cholesterol, triglycerides, and aerobic fitness with the subjects most available to me: out-of-shape college students. What I found opened my eyes: Doing exercise that barely broke a sweat was just as good as a high-intensity run. It got me thinking that perhaps we don't have to break our backs to get fit and healthy.

But there is a trade-off. We might not have to break out in a sweat to see results, but we'd have to exercise for a much longer period of time. It's a reality: The greatest return on an exercise investment definitely comes with more vigorous workouts. But both these suppositions had built-in problems for sedentary people. They wouldn't want to work out any longer than they'd have to. Nor would they want to exercise at an intensity that would leave them crumpled on the floor.

That's when my Spark ignited: *What if the exercise that people did was intense enough to give them all the benefits of vigorous activity— but not so long in duration that it was next to impossible to fit into a normal person's schedule?*

Could it be done?

I began to refocus on my experience with professional athletes. World-class endurance athletes, especially runners, weight-lifters, and swimmers, always divided their daily workouts into shorter segments. Instead of running a full 20 miles a day, for example, they might run 7 miles in the morning, 5 around midday, and 8 in the late afternoon. By breaking up their workouts, they weren't worn down. They remained strong. It gave them an edge over the competition.

If it worked for world-class athletes, why not for everyone?

It was time to take my theories to the street. If college students, in their prime, could find significant health and fitness improvements within three weeks, what about people my own age, graying baby boomers who might not have seen the inside of a gym since high school? Could I help *them* become healthier?

The Spark study gave me the answer: a resounding yes.

It is quite possible to reverse years, even decades, of sedentary abuse—within three weeks.

K's Spark

My family's "Spark" had nothing to do with physical exercise. Oh, they had a zest for living, all right, as long as they could get there by car. My dad had a large hunger for knowledge and people. And, unfortunately, a seemingly bottomless hunger for food and drink as well. Eating was our pastime, our joy of life. Graduate college? Eat a pound cake. Get a job in your major? Wine and cheese. Sunday night get-together? Thick steaks and hot-fudge sundaes or take-out Chinese food.

It's how I grew up, what I knew. Except when it came to using my mind, exercise was as foreign to me as finger bowls and dressing for dinner. I was sedentary from the neck down.

When my father died of a sudden heart attack at fifty-two, we called it a terrible twist of fate. It didn't occur to me that my family history was rich in risk. Cholesterol was a strange-sounding word found in scientific journals. I kept going the way I knew best. I found solace (and love, comfort, joy, and relief) in food throughout my life. I even ate while I wrote.

Here I was in Mesa Verde unable to breathe, when it hit me as hard as a frozen quart of Chunky Monkey: My family had heart disease. All of us.

But what could I do? I couldn't just bounce back with a crash liquid diet or another aerobics class. I couldn't think past the strain of putting on a plus-size leotard.

I had a headache. I felt overwhelmed. I was fat. I was out of *shape. So what if I was a good person? A good wife? A good daughter? I was still going to die too soon. I looked up at D.J. and smiled. "I need to eat."*

From the start, the scientist in me plunged into the complexities of the Spark almost to the exclusion of everything else. I went to sleep thinking about muscular strength and aerobic capacity, or an element of metabolic efficiency that needed to be explored. In researching an unrelated topic in my office, I'd find myself going off on a Spark tangent about fiber. I talked about the Spark so much at home that my family began to tease me.

And then there were the people:

Dianne V. came up the gymnasium complex stairs at the University of Virginia huffing and puffing. She walked into my office pretending she wasn't out of breath, trying to smile and say hello. Dianne was thirty-eight and weighed 235 pounds. Heart disease ran in her family and she didn't want to have to take medication later on in life. She'd asked to be a part of the Spark because she'd tried every diet out there and always gained back the weight she'd initially lost. As she was approaching her forties, she realized that she had to take better care of her health, which meant regular, consistent exercise, something she'd never done before. She told me she wanted to be able to walk up the stairs carrying her backpack without having to stop every few steps.

Pat S. was five years older, and her goals were similar. At forty-three, she wanted to have more energy to raise her two children, hold down a full-time job, and, whenever she could fit it in, enjoy her personal time more. She certainly didn't want to spend the hour or so she had after the kids were asleep exercising. It felt like work to squeeze exercise in when she was exhausted. Until she joined the study, she didn't know she had any other option.

Joanne H., age fifty, wanted to be the best participant in the study. She came on board ready to soar. She was sick and tired of being out of shape. "I refuse to age gracefully."

Mary W. had a beautiful face, with the sculpted cheekbones of a queen. During the preliminary testing she learned she had a body fat index that was only slightly above average for her age of forty-two. Mary wanted to lose weight, but she was realistic. After having three children, she knew she'd never be thin. But healthy, toned, and strong was another matter.

Each of the forty participants in the study approached the Spark with the same combination of trepidation and excitement, resolve and skepticism they'd approached other programs with. But there was something more here, something fundamentally different. I could feel it and they could feel it.

The Spark spoke to them, to their lifestyles and needs. Even more important, it made sense in the context of their lives.

When I first put the word out for the Spark study, I assumed I'd get a few responses—if I was lucky. But within two days, my e-mail was filled with notes from people eager to try out the program. Most of them were out of shape or had gone in and out of exercise programs throughout their adult lives. They were aging baby boomers, men and women, some as young as thirty-two, others as old as sixty-eight. Some had high cholesterol or stiff joints or trouble getting up the stairs. Others lacked the energy to get through their day without a struggle. And still others were fairly healthy and wanted only to get rid of their middle-age bulge. But one common thread tied them all together: a desire to be fit and trim. Strong. Healthy. Brimming with possibilities.

The Spark was catching fire.

The forty people in the initial Spark study filled out lifestyle questionnaires similar to the ones you'll use in this book. They spent a half hour performing tests that evaluated their fitness, strength-training capability, and flexibility (exactly like the ones you'll be doing to get you started on the Spark). They also had their blood analyzed at the university laboratory. (You won't be able to get a blood analysis unless you go to your doctor, but I've formulated a short test for this book to give you a general idea of your heart and blood health.)

Armed with their initial numbers, the group was eager to Spark. And Spark they did for three weeks—instead of three months. They built up to a total of 15 ten-minute exercise Sparks a week (divided into a specific number of aerobic, strength-training, and flexibility Sparks determined by the results of their tests).

Some of the people in the study walked around the block.

Some of them walked on treadmills at home.

Some of them lifted weights in their offices.

Some of them did stretches before they went to sleep.

Some of them danced to music in their living rooms.

And, of the initial forty people in the group, *all of them stayed on the Spark*—and were ready for more after the three weeks ended.

They were motivated, not only because they could now easily fit exercise into their daily lives, but because of a newfound vigor and strength. On average, in only three weeks:

- Aerobic capacity improved by 10 to 15 percent, the equivalent fitness level of a person *ten to fifteen years younger.*
- Strength and muscular endurance improved from 40 percent to 100 percent, to the equivalent strength level of a person *twenty years younger.*
- Flexibility scores increased to the equivalent range of motion of *someone younger by twenty years.*

- Weight loss averaged 3 pounds; *a consistent, healthy start of about 1 pound a week.*
- Total cholesterol dropped 15 points in the group as a whole—and by 34 points in those participants in the high-risk range. A 1 percent reduction in cholesterol reduces heart disease risk by 3 percent. *This means that the average Spark study participant reduced their risk of heart disease by 20 percent*—and those in the high-risk range reduced their risk by close to 40 percent!
- LDL or "bad" cholesterol dropped 10 points in the group as a whole—and 29 points for those in the high-risk range. *And everyone who started the study in the high-risk category got out of it!*
- Triglyceride levels decreased from 120 points to 96—about a *20 percent decrease in three weeks.*

The numbers speak for themselves. The Spark was more than "catching fire" now. It had become a flame.

K's Spark

I wish I could say that my horrendous climb up the Mesa Verde hills was a starting point for my new life, that it was a completely conscious progression from that heart-stopping tour to the Boston–New York AIDS Ride, the 275-mile three-day bike trek I completed two years later. But it wasn't. To be honest, I didn't even realize what I was doing. I just put my feet to the pedals and ignored everything else. The slogan for the Boston–New York AIDS Ride says it best: "Our greatest fear is not that we are inadequate. Our greatest fear is that we are powerful beyond measure."

Maybe you once had a metabolism that never seemed to quit. Energy that kept you going when a deadline was near and the ability to dance all night and come back for more.

But somewhere along the way, you lost it. Perhaps your doctor put you on medication for elevated cholesterol; she told you your blood pressure was too high and your triglycerides were going through the roof. Perhaps you learned that you were diabetic, and your future looked gray—and tasteless. Perhaps the signs were more subtle: You stopped running up the stairs when you forgot something. You started taking your car to go to the market—one block away. You not only yearned to take a nap in the middle of the afternoon, you *needed* one to stay awake for an evening out.

Do not despair. Your Spark is still there, waiting, like embers in a fire to become a flame. Like so many of the people in the Spark study at the University of Virginia, and like Karla, the steadfast couch potato on the cliffs of Mesa Verde, you too can rekindle your Spark. You too can lower your cholesterol, reduce your blood pressure, keep blood sugar levels within a healthy range, and reignite the feeling of health you once had. You too can lose excess weight, tone your body, and feel incredibly energetic—at any age.

This isn't an empty promise. This is a reality. And all you need to make your own Spark a soaring flame is . . . a Spark, a quick burst of exercise, ten minutes total. Combined with the Spark healthy diet eating plan, you'll not only steadily improve your health and the way you look but nearly every single aspect of your life, imbuing your mind, body, and soul with confidence, strength, and vigor.

All you need is three weeks to see results. And *that* is a concrete, thoroughly documented, scientifically and medically sound guarantee.

THE SPARK

K's Spark

Within these pages, you'll learn what I did—and didn't do—to change my life during the two years after my ultimately fortuitous Mesa Verde climb. It wasn't easy; when is it ever? We all know some things die hard. Among them for me were my passion for carbs, television, and a reclining position. I was in the midst of all three when I happened to see Glenn talking about fitness on TV on the February 16, 1999, edition of *Dateline*. I put down my bowl of cereal and stared at the tube. "Ohmigod. This is me. This man is talking to me."

The next day, I tracked Glenn down at the University of Virginia and, after assuring him I wasn't some crazed stalker, talked to him about writing a book together.

This book was born that February, with Glenn as the authority and I as inspiration: a middle-aged, overweight, at-risk couch potato who, by following her version of the Spark, had become an athlete and fitness instructor, I literally and figuratively changed my life; I lost forty-five pounds and dropped my triglycerides, blood pressure, and cholesterol.

Within these pages, you'll find everything you need to rekindle your health, your looks, and your life.

You'll begin your three-week journey with a complete understanding of the Spark: what it is, how it works, and *why* it works. Myths are exposed. Possibility becomes promise.

Next come the quizzes, the important—and entertaining—preliminary testing that determines where and how you start the Spark. You'll find simple ways to discover your . . .

. . . potential "bad" body fat (what really is unhealthy and what is just fine);

. . . fitness level (so you'll have the right combination of aerobic, strength-training, and flexibility Sparks to light your flame);

. . . appetite IQ (as you become aware of your true sense of fullness);

. . . exercise personality (and custom-design your activity program, Sparking to your own music at your own time).

After you've gotten to know yourself and your individual Spark possibilities, you're ready to begin. The next section of the book provides the actual program: what you need to do and how to do it, week by week.

Week One: Embers. Time to move, but only for a few minutes at a time. This is the week to begin incorporating exercise into your life: strength training, flexibility, and aerobics.

Week Two: Kindling. You're building up to 10-minute Sparks, 15 times a week. Depending on the results of your Spark tests, some of you will be concentrating on strength, some of you on flexibility and range of motion, and others of you on getting that heart pumping stronger.

Week Three: The Fire and Beyond. The Spark program for the rest of your life, the 10-minute equation for health, vitality, and good looks, too.

But a fire, whether an ember or a fiery blaze, needs fuel to stay lit. Your body, too, needs fuel, a strong, steady metabolism to keep it going, and that's where the Spark Food Plan comes in. If you diet without exercise, your fire may get the right fuel, but it won't stay lit. You won't be stoking that fire efficiently. Eventually, the fire will be put out; you'll become sluggish and listless. Too much "junk quality" fuel and the fire won't ignite at all. You need the right balance of fuel, the right amount of stoking *all day long,* to make that healthy burn, to make your body strong and revved up.

The Spark Food Plan, the culmination of my years of research and study into the most effective way to burn calories, uses an exact, built-in equation with three components:

Spark Fuel (SF). The food you eat each day, especially complex carbohydrate–rich meals and snacks (including cereals, rice, whole grain breads, pasta, beans, fruits, vegetables—even nuts, bran muffins, and the ubiquitous bagel).

Spark Burn (SB). The ideal place where what you eat and what you burn combine, promoting health, vitality, and weight loss.

And the element that keeps your **SF-SB** Flame alive?

Spark Fiber. The more fruits, vegetables, and grains you eat, the more effective your **SF-SB** equation will be. And the more efficient your body is, the stronger and fitter you'll feel and the more weight you'll lose.

You'll find the foods you need for vitality and health in the Basic Spark Food Plan in Chapter 5.

Along with one full week of Spark food menu plans, I've provided exercise plans, 10-minute Sparks, for you to do. These sample exercise plans are tailored to your specific stage on your Spark journey and include two Embers, two Kindlings, and three Fires (see Appendix A).

As you begin the Spark you'll also find some exciting surprises:

- The Spark way of exercising also promotes an infusion of growth hormone—that "fountain of youth" that usually decreases as you age.

- Fueling your Spark means getting your pasta back—and eating it too. Bagels. Bananas. Baked potatoes and corn. Despite the recent bad press starches have received, carbs, especially those packed with fiber, mean health. In fact, researchers at the University of Pittsburgh School of Medicine conducted a nationwide study that tracked people of all ages who have been on diets—and found that **those who were most successful at maintaining their weight loss ate a high-carbohydrate diet.**

You'll also find:

- Strategies to get an exercise Spark in at lunchtime without the sweat.
- Easy, fast, and efficient 10-minute Spark sessions that include warm-up and cool-down time!
- A routine of important weight-resistance training and stretching that was used successfully in the Spark study at the University of Virginia. *Not in addition to your 15 weekly Sparks, but as part of them.*
- Definitive proof from the participants in the Spark study that these 15 Sparks, done anywhere, at any time, without special knowledge, equipment, or a great deal of motivation, will rev up your metabolism, balance your insulin levels, lower your risk of heart disease, and get rid of excess weight—all within three weeks!

Think of the total package: 10-minute Sparks of exercise that help you lose body fat and look younger, keep your metabolism high, your cardiovascular system healthy, your bones and muscles strong, and your mind alert combined with an easy-to-manage eating plan that promises the carbs you love.

Are you ready to Spark?

CHAPTER 2

Why the Spark?

In 1814, rehearsals of Beethoven's Seventh Symphony began—the culmination of bits of paper, pencil sketches, and notebooks the composer created, so the legend goes, then tossed into the corner of his room. The amount of time Beethoven spent on his sketchbooks? Less than 10 minutes at a time.

THE SPARK AS A WHOLE NEW WAY OF LOOKING AT EXERCISE

Hear the word *exercise* and, if you're like most people, you'll conjure up images of heavy gym bags, sweaty clothes, crowded classes blaring the latest rock hit, and the big rush to change, shower, and get back to your life. Exercise is something separate from your life, something you have to do, something you have to fit in. *Wrong!* **The Spark's 10-minute bursts of activity two or three times a day can be more effective for both health and weight management than a traditional workout at the gym—and easier to maintain over the long term.**

SPARK PLUG

On February 22, 2000, the American Heart Association Science Advisory Committee published the results of its review of resistance-training exercises on the development of muscular strength and endurance. The findings? Performing moderate- to high-intensity resistance training 2 to 3 days a week over a period of 3 to 6 months will improve muscular strength and endurance by 35 percent to 100 percent in both men and women of all ages. **The Spark Study 2000 shows exactly the same results in only 3 weeks.**

A Spark is *not* running into your kids' rooms to get them ready for school or 10 minutes of rushing through your morning routine because you're late. It *is* a completely researched, tested, and specific burst of activity that has been found to be the most lifestyle-friendly way to get fit and trim—and stay that way.

The numbers speak for themselves. The results of my Spark study unequivocally show a *10 to 15 percent improvement in aerobic fitness among middle-aged men and women.* These are the same results (and in some cases even greater) that I found in my studies of younger athletes using traditional training approaches of long, once-a-day exercise sessions.

The January 27, 1999 issue of the *Journal of the American Medical Association (JAMA)* reinforced the conclusions of my latest work in the published findings of a study done at the Department of Geriatric Medicine at the Johns Hopkins Medical School. This particular study found a major "secret" for weight maintenance: an active lifestyle. No surprise here, but wait: It also found that incorporating lifestyle Sparks (short bursts of activity) is as effective for improving health and fitness in previously sedentary adults as a structured, steadfast 45 minutes three times a week exercise regime. Even more telling: These results occurred after a 4- to 16-month period. *My data showed the same results in only three weeks.*

The researchers at Johns Hopkins also found that people who did lifestyle Sparks throughout the day consistently lost weight, and they found that these *lifestyle Sparks were more effective at keeping weight off for good.* People who did traditional "45/3" exercise sessions combined with a 16-week diet program ended up gaining 25 percent of their weight back one year later, *but the group who continued to do lifestyle Sparks did not gain!* One year later, they had maintained their healthy weight.

In total, you'll need only 15 Sparks a week to:

- Improve aerobic and metabolic fitness
- Strengthen muscle endurance and increase flexibility
- Reduce excess body fat

SPARKLER

"When I contacted you with a 'Yes, I want to participate,' I was really unsure as to whether I could physically commit to the routine. But after realizing that every exercise you suggested was something that I could do, I really liked the idea. I found the program definitely beneficial in getting me started exercising. I feel much more flexible, my back and shoulders are not nearly as stressed when I sit for hours at the computer, and I am able to get into a size smaller in my clothes."

—BRENDA M., a fifty-two-year-old office manager

- Lower your cholesterol
- Keep your triglycerides in check
- Consistently lose the pounds that count—not water weight and not lean muscle tissue
- Reduce muscle and joint aches and pains
- Become more energetic and vital
- Sleep better than you have in years

Think of it: **15 10-minute bursts of activity, or just 2½ hours of Sparks a week, is all you need to feel and look great!**

These 15 10-minute Sparks consist of aerobic bursts to work your heart and lungs, complemented with simple, easy-to-follow strength-training and flexibility/stretching routines. These Sparks are exactly like the ones used in the University of Virginia study and have specifically been chosen for their fast results and portability. You'll find the specifics of the Spark Exercise Plan—and how to create your own individual plan—in Chapters 3 and 4.

Put another way, you can rekindle your health, your looks, and your life with only 15 Sparks a week. For most of you, the "Spark equation" will be:

- 7 to 10 aerobic Sparks (which include warm-up and cool-down)
- 2 to 4 strength-training Sparks (to keep muscles strong and bones healthy)
- 2 to 4 flexibility Sparks (yoga-like stretches you can do in between meetings, carpools, or before you go to sleep)

With the Spark, you no longer have to make an effort to "fit in your exercise." You can forget long, arduous exercise sessions. You don't have to plan your day, pack a gym bag, or push yourself mentally or physically to make exercise a part of your life.

K's Spark

It's hard work to stop thinking a certain way or to admit something isn't working, not because you weren't good enough, or smart enough, or talented enough, but because you chose the wrong vehicle to get there.

Take exercise for example. What is it about that concept that makes it such a big deal for people? Well, I know what it was for me. The Commitment. The Time. The Equipment. The "Shoulds." It's no wonder that even before I tied my first sneaker before exercising, I was exhausted. I'd scoff at the magazine articles that actually implied that exercise was fun. Fun? Who actually enjoyed hunkering down with a 10-pound dumbbell? To me, exercise was all work.

After all, it was ingrained in me, by everyone from my phys ed teacher to my internist, to the countless diets I tried and the health clubs I joined: get your heart rate up for at least 20 minutes at a time, three to five times a week. If I missed a session, which invariably would happen, I'd feel so bad I'd eat a piece of cake.

But the one thing I learned as I continued to find my Spark was that before you can have fun, you do have to work hard—not at jumping, running, or tying a sneaker, but at changing the way you think.

I had to change the way my mind worked. I simply had no choice but to let go of my old ways. And let me tell you: Once you do let go, there's an overwhelming sense of relief. The "shoulds" melt away like fat-free sorbet and, in their place, dare I say, is fun.

What took me so long?

STAYING YOUNG:
THE SPARK AND GROWTH HORMONE

The Spark is much more than a diet and exercise program—and it literally changes the way you age. A "fountain of youth" hormone has been found to be released during exercise, not just while training for a triathlon or taking kickboxing classes back-to-back, but by *simply walking at a brisk pace for as little as 10 minutes* or riding your bike to the park on a glorious Sunday afternoon or dancing to a favorite song

---

SPARK PLUG

In 1995, *The International Journal of Obesity* reported on a study involving two groups of overweight women in their forties. One group of women did 10 minutes of Spark-type exercises two to four times a day, the other group exercised just once a day for 20 to 40 minutes. The results? *The "Spark" group not only stuck better to their exercise program, they also lost an average of 20 pounds—6 more pounds than the "once a day" group.* In 1997, the same research team performed a similar study for the same journal. This time around *they also discovered that those women in the worst shape, with poor fitness levels, high body fat, and high insulin levels, improved the most when on a Spark-like program.*

Just ask Dianne V., one of the participants in the Spark Study 2000. She not only got her cholesterol levels out of the high-risk range, with 90 percent of the drop in LDL, or "bad" cholesterol, but *she also lost 26 pounds in three weeks on the Spark plan.*

It's never too late to start the Spark.

---

on the radio. Nothing that will make you break out in a profuse sweat (but will give you an attractive glow!). Nothing that a tried-and-true couch potato can't do. Ten minutes two or three times a day, on most days of the week: in the morning, perhaps, when going out to get your paper before breakfast, during your lunch break at the office, and when you get home, either before or after dinner. *Ten minutes, two or three times a day.* That's all you need to tap into your very own "fountain of youth."

As we age and put on weight, we lose our ability to produce and secrete growth hormone (GH), which, in our youth, made our bones strong, our bodies supple, our immune system hearty. GH can seemingly "turn back the clock." GH injections are available, but only to the rich. As an anti-aging serum, it's expensive at best and a danger to your health at worst. With the right kind of activity, *three times a day, your own body is stimulated once again to release this hormone,* naturally. *Safely.* In fact, recent research on GH and exercise conducted at the University of Virginia indicates that multiple bursts of exercise—the Spark way of exercise—pack the most wallop.

Your body is continually producing and secreting GH when you exercise for short bouts (Sparks!) a few times a day. But when you exercise only once a day, your body compensates, slowing down the GH secretions—regardless of how long that exercise session may be. In the same way your metabolism shuts down when you starve yourself on a stringent diet, GH goes into slow motion. Your body feels the need to conserve its valuable surge of GH and, as the day goes on, you get less and less output. In other words, you might *think* you're turning back the clock when you push yourself through a 45-minute Tae-Bo class, but, in reality, you're going to be secreting less and less GH throughout the day. (If you're a die-hard exercise enthusiast, you might find this hard to believe, but it is true. Studies have shown that

---

SPARKLER

"Short exercise segments are the reality of my life. I don't have the time to do more. So the fact that this works is great! I feel better, I lost weight, and my cholesterol is lower. The Spark proves to me that less is more."

—MARY W., editorial assistant and mother of three

---

the more intermittent activity you do, the more spurts of GH you produce. If you're spending 45 minutes in the gym and that's it for the day, your body compensates later—by producing and secreting *less* GH!) If you only did a couple of easy kickboxing moves throughout the day (10-minute kicks three times a day!), you'd actually keep yourself younger—longer.

THE SPARK THAT LINGERS: BURNING CALORIES IN YOUR SLEEP

Imagine a metabolism that wakes up so much that you have a metabolic "afterburn" that *may last for days* after only one day of short, active Sparks. This afterburn makes your body more effective in metabolizing the food you eat. In addition to burning more calories, your body won't need as much insulin to help process your food—and you'll lower your triglyceride levels to boot. In fact, you'll be revving up your metabolism enough by doing only 15 Sparks a week on the program that you can skip a couple of days and still get a metabolic "high."

An even better metabolic side effect: A day of exercise Sparks helps

---

SPARK PLUG

In 1998, the prestigious *Medicine & Science in Sports & Exercise* published a study from the United Kingdom's Loughborough University that compared two different exercise styles on women in their forties **over a period of three months.** One group of women walked briskly for 30 uninterrupted minutes a day; the other group walked briskly for only 10 minutes, three times a day. Both groups walked at an intensity that ensured a good cardiovascular workout, and both groups achieved equal aerobic capacity improvements. *But the women who walked in brief 10-minute bursts lost close to twice as much weight as the "30 minutes once a day" group. The Spark-like group also showed other considerable improvements: a 70 percent greater reduction of waist size and a 60 percent greater drop in blood pressure.*

The Spark Study 2000 showed these same results in weight loss and cardiovascular fitness, not in three months, *but in only three weeks.*

---

decrease your appetite, making your diet Sparks that much more effective. In fact, a 1995 study at the University of Pittsburgh School of Medicine demonstrated that women who did Spark-like exercise lost more weight than women who did more traditional modes of exercise. The results showed that doing *Spark-like exercise for 10 minutes three times a day reduced daily caloric intake by 140 calories*—which equals a whopping 50,000 calories per year!

THE SPARK FOOD PLAN:
CARBOHYDRATES CAN MAKE YOU SLIMMER

Just as your exercise Sparks are different from other regimes, so are your food Sparks. The Spark Food Plan is not based on bizarre food combinations, strict caloric restrictions, and eating time constraints. It's not based on taboo foods, sending imaginary food police to inspect your cupboards for illegal pastas, crackers, or rice. It's not based on high-protein dogma, spreading the erroneous message that protein—fat, lean, or fried—is the only way to go.

The Spark diet is based on fuel. Yes, fuel. Not necessarily sexy or trendy, but tried, true, and necessary for life.

Quite simply, food is fuel. The more you exercise, the more fuel you need. The more you burn calories, the more food you need to stoke the fire. Everyone knows that old axiom "The only way to lose weight is to expend more calories than you consume." Exercise burns calories and builds muscle—and muscles burn more calories than fat. In fact, for every pound of muscle you build, you burn about 10 more calories every day. This might not seem like a lot, but 10 calories a day comes to 3,500 calories per year.

The most efficient way to burn these calories? Exercise—*and eating fiber-rich carbohydrates.* With your body fine-tuned, metabolically efficient, and strong from your exercise Sparks, that tempting bowl of pasta or beckoning banana won't make you fat. Exercise is the trigger. Exercise changes food. Pasta, bananas, rice, big round bagels—none of them will make you gain weight. Exercise becomes diet, a way to manage weight.

In other words, doing your 10-minute exercise Sparks means you can and *should* eat complex carbohydrates to lose weight and feel fit.

SPARK PLUG

An August 1999 Gallup Poll found that 40 percent of those people who followed a high-protein, low-carbohydrate diet gained their weight back. *But only 15 percent of Spark-like dieters, with its emphasis on complex carbohydrates, gained back their pounds.* **You might lose weight on a high-protein diet, but the pounds won't stay off.**

That's correct. Carbohydrates. Starch. Those supposedly "evil" foods that are bad for mind and body. Despite the bad press starches have received, carbs, especially those packed with fiber, mean health. Studies show that *peak-performing athletes consistently eat carbohydrates* to give them energy and help them lose excess weight.

And yet, despite the scientific evidence, the medical proof, that carbohydrates are vital for healthy weight management, many of us continue to spurn them:

"I know my own body. And I can't eat bread."

"I get bloated when I eat carbohydrates."

"I couldn't lose weight until I cut out carbs."

Sound familiar? I've attempted to analyze the reasons that people, from celebrities to journalists, housewives to stockbrokers, people from all walks of life, continue to praise high-protein diets and condemn breads and other starches.

It can't be because they work. They don't. These high-protein diets have been around for more than forty years. If they worked, we'd be a nation of thin people. Instead, we're fatter than ever.

I think the answer lies in a combination of chemistry, myth, history, psychology—and a whole lot of wishful thinking.

Chemical Reaction. Low-carbohydrate diets use the analogy of fattening up cattle and pigs with carbs and grains. No argument here. Animals quickly synthesize fat from these carbohydrates (think of the well-known phrase "corn-fed pigs"); that's how they are fattened up. (It doesn't hurt that they lead pretty sedentary lives either.) At first glance, this one might sound plausible. Until you remember that humans are not cattle—or pigs. We have a very poor capacity for converting dietary carbohydrates into fat. When humans overeat a mix of calories, the carbs are preferentially burned while the dietary fat goes straight into fat cells. There's a biochemical continent between us and our four-legged friends. But we hear the analogy and find it compelling; it sounds right, even though it's wrong.

Ancient Greece. Our attraction to proteins stems back to ancient times. It was on the Greek islands that protein was first discovered to be vital for health. Indeed, the word *protein* is taken from the Greek word *protos,* meaning "first importance." Hundreds of years after those Hellenic days, protein is still associated with muscles, with lean, powerful bodies. And, yes, muscles contain protein, and the bigger the muscles, the more protein is synthesized in the body. But there's a big leap between the protein found in the muscles in the body and actually *eating* protein. One doesn't translate to the other.

Snob Appeal. Carbohydrates represent cheap food. Dishes made with protein and fat are more expensive; pasta is always the cheaper entrée on the menu. You can always find cheap food; boxes of convenience items such as macaroni, snack bars, and cereals proliferate on grocery store shelves throughout the world. But fresh foods, crisp greens, lean meats, and nouveau cuisine are a lot more expensive—and a lot less convenient.

There is a certain snobbery associated with your eating arugula and a veal chop while your neighbor eats macaroni and cheese.

The Psychology of Sin. One of the Seven Deadly Sins is gluttony. Combine gluttony with our puritanical roots, and you have a classic power struggle between virtue and indulgence. In order to lose weight, you have to feel deprived. And what better way to deprive yourself than pushing away a plate of pasta, a slice of warm, crusty bread, a thick, fresh bagel? Unfortunately, this "dieting is deprivation" way of thinking leads to bingeing and other eating disorders when indulgence wins the struggle.

Tricking Fate. You know fat makes you fat. You hate what fat can do to your body. You also know that some fat is artery clogging and dense with the possibility of excess weight. And, yet, here you are eating all the fat that you want—without any of it settling on your body. It's sinful, delicious, daring. Eat fat and get thin. Much sexier than rice. But can you really cheat Nature?

Misinformation. The number one item people cut out when they start a diet is sweets. Candy, desserts, and other confectioneries are associated with calories, blood sugar swings, even weakness of character. Unfortunately, many Americans connect carbohydrates with sweets. True, sugar is a carbohydrate, but there is a difference between healthy complex carbohydrates and simple, refined sugars. Pecan pie is not the same as granola. A croissant is not the same as a bran muffin. Ice cream is not the same as a plate of pasta. But many people equate the two, believing that starch is sugar, and sugar, starch. In reality, carbohydrates themselves don't make you fat. It's the fat you add that makes you, well, you know the rest. . . .

Still not ready to give yourself permission to eat a bagel in the morning and pasta primavera at night? Think globally. If you take the world's population and graph the relationship between relative body weight and carbohydrate intake, you'll see *that people who eat more carbs weigh less*. In rural China, for example, farmers consume several hundred calories more per day than Americans, many of those calories from rice—a carbohydrate. Yet obesity in rural China is *virtually nonexistent*. These farmers conform to the way our "hunter-gatherer" bodies were initially designed and evolved: "grazing" or nibbling food throughout the day, while at the same time performing frequent bouts of necessary activity—the hunting and gathering needed to sustain life. These rural Chinese, and other more simple-living peoples across the globe, instinctively live the fat-burning, energy-fueling Spark way of life that we need to rekindle: a *healthful*, high-carbohydrate diet combined with short bursts of strategically timed exercise. (Another plus for all that rice: Heart disease is virtually nonexistent in rural China. Americans are twenty times more likely to have a heart attack than their Asian counterparts.)

It's difficult to put aside the promise of rapid weight loss in high-protein diets, and the "carbs make you fat" mentality, but the facts

---

SPARK PLUG

A 1993 study published in the *American Journal of Clinical Nutrition* found that insulin levels stayed even and "bad" LDL cholesterol levels decreased when people shunned the standard "three square" meals and, instead, ate the same calories in smaller, multiple meals—the "nibbling" way of eating on the Spark Food Plan.

SPARKLER

"It's not like you're really dieting on the Spark plan. So you don't have to make an effort to think about what you're eating and how much. All I did was add more fiber to my diet. I never felt hungry!"

—PAT S., Spark study participant and
licensed real estate broker

---

speak for themselves—as do the results of studies, such as those ongoing at the University of Virginia and those completed and published in the most prestigious journals of our day.

THE SPARK FOOD PLAN:
A NEW WAY OF EATING FOR LIFE

Carbohydrates are only part of the story. Like the ease and convenience of your Spark exercises, your Spark foods are also "easy to swallow." In fact, there are no rules but one: eat fiber. You'll be eating healthier and more efficiently with extra fiber (as in those infamous carbs!) on the Spark plan—reaching a goal in three weeks of 25 grams of fiber a day.

If the idea of simply adding fiber to your diet to lose weight sounds implausible, think again. A comprehensive ten-year study of nearly 3,000 men and women, published in the *Journal of the American Medical Association* in 1999, found that those **people who consumed the most fiber had the best success in controlling their weight—**

regardless of the amount of calories they consumed. The people who gained the most weight? *Those who ate a low-fat, low-fiber diet.* In other words, high fiber is the answer to weight control—not simply lowering your fat intake.

The Spark Food Plan, with its emphasis on high-fiber carbohydrates, will give you that weight control boost you need and, as an added plus, *naturally* prevent you from eating too much fat. High-fiber carbs are more satiating than other foods; they add bulk to your diet and you're less likely to feel hungry after a meal. As John Blundell, an internationally recognized "appetite expert," and his colleagues reported in a 1999 article in the *International Journal of Food Sciences & Nutrition*, eating a high-fiber, carbohydrate-rich breakfast creates a feeling of fullness that helps maintain weight loss.

More good news about fiber: A 1997 report by researchers at the United States Department of Agriculture found that fiber is a fat magnet, grabbing on to the fat in ingested food and preventing your body from absorbing it. The average American eats only about 12 to 15 grams of fiber daily. If you merely double that fiber intake (simply by eating a couple of pieces of fruit and two slices of whole grain bread), your body would be prevented from absorbing approximately 32,000 calories a year. This translates into 8 pounds of fat that isn't absorbed. In other words, it's possible to lose 8 pounds in a year if you do nothing but sprinkle extra bran on your yogurt, switch to multigrain bread, and eat a peach or an apple as an additional snack every day. *(The Spark Food Plan will show you how to easily switch to high-fiber alternatives—without adding extra calories.)* An added plus: eating an additional two pieces of fruit and an extra two slices of whole grain bread every day (which equals about 12 to 15 grams of fiber) can reduce your risk of heart disease by more than 40 percent—*no matter what you weigh!*

K's Spark

I'd read in a woman's magazine that diets are most successful in people who have good body images to begin with. No kidding. But here's the irony: if you have a good body image, there's no need to diet. The motivation, the "I'm too fat and I have to do something about it," isn't there.

However, for those of us with a poor body image, like me, it's another story. Of course, I wasn't born hating my stomach or my thighs. I didn't lie in my crib thinking I was too fat. My love-hate relationship with my body image began about forty-five years ago, when I was walking to school one morning in the sixth grade. A group of kids were behind me, kids I knew, kids I saw every day and even played with in the afternoons. They were mumbling, their voices growing in pitch as we got closer to the crossing guard. "Hey, look at that hippopotamus go." "Fatty." "Oink. Oink." I looked around. Who were they talking about?

The only other kid I saw near the corner was Beth. She was red-haired, freckled, and stick thin. There was Janice, of course, my best friend, but she was walking with me. She and I borrowed each other's clothes all the time and I wasn't fat, so she couldn't be.

While we all waited for the traffic to ease, the name-calling grew worse. They were pointing at me. Wait a minute. They were talking about me! I was the hippo.

That image has stayed with me for the past forty years. I was big and fat and nothing could change that: not a compliment, a marriage proposal, a promotion on the job. Not even being thin.

Diets—and going off them—became my modus operandi. I became a muffin vigilante, a secret cereal eater in the middle of the night. My body image went from poor to worse and no diet in the world seemed to make a difference.

Maybe, contradictory as it seemed, dieting was wrong—at least the gimmicky, deprivation-oriented way I was going about it. Rather than use my mouth, I used my legs.

I knew if I could ride a bike, swim a lap, dance a tango, I would feel better about myself. That poor body image would vanish— and in its place would be an active, healthy woman who didn't need to be super thin.

Exercise could be my diet. And there would be no looking back.

THE SPARK FUEL–SPARK BURN EQUATION FOR WEIGHT CONTROL

Close your eyes for a moment and imagine yourself sitting in front of a campfire. The fire is roaring, the flames leaping up into the night sky. It seems as if the blaze would soar forever as you stare into the fire, but, of course, the flames are only as strong as the logs they feed on. Eventually, as the logs are burned, the flames become subdued; the wood is almost used up. You need to throw some more logs onto the fire, to bring it back to life. But not just any logs. Wet or sap-laden wood isn't going to burn; crisp dry wood is best. Nor is simply piling on the wood enough, even if it is nice and dry. Without oxygen, the fire will continue to dim until it goes out. The wood has to be stoked and turned and pushed about. You not only need to add the right fuel, you need to move it around.

This campfire, the wood and its movement, is similar to the way your body consumes food and burns calories—and it is less of a stretch than you might think. If you stop eating, your fire will go out. (This is one of the reasons why starvation diets don't work. Your metabolism slows down so much in order to conserve energy that you end up losing less and less weight.)

If you eat too much of the wrong thing (think of sweets and fats as wet, sap-laden wood), the fire won't stay strong. It just won't burn off the calories.

And if you don't move your body, you just won't burn enough of that fuel to lose excess weight.

You need just the right balance between the fuel you put in and the calories that you expend in order to keep your fire burning. And thanks to the Spark plan, that perfect balance is achieved. The food and exercise Sparks work synergistically, each empowering the other, in a relationship similar to starting and maintaining that soaring nighttime campfire.

Spark Fuel, or **SF,** is the logs, the fuel that gets your fire going. The foods you eat, specifically your body's primary fuel sources, carbohydrates and fats, will determine the strength of your flames, as well as the ability of your fire to "take" easily and well.

High-fiber carbohydrates are like those crisp, dry logs. Your muscles take to them like a sponge, grabbing them and utilizing them as fuel. Because you're consuming less fat, most of the carbs go right to the muscles and are used up quickly—either burned as fuel or stored for your next round of exercise. The rest of your body, hungry for the carbs your muscles grabbed, must then turn around and look for something else to "eat": the fat you have stored on your body. Suddenly, the fat that's been hanging around all this time is being used. Burned up. Gone up in smoke.

If you eat a high-fiber, high-carb diet as in the Spark Food Plan, you'll *naturally* eat less fat because you'll be fuller faster and longer—

which means your body will, by necessity, be burning those carbs—and heading toward that stored fat for more food. You'll have a high **SF**—*the ideal place for weight loss and weight control.*

If, on the other hand, you eat a lot of fatty foods but few carbs, your body will only eat the just ingested fat. You'll never get around to the fat in those stored fat cells; there's too much, too convenient, "fresh fodder." You'll have a low **SF,** which will ultimately put your weight back on (and then some).

Spark Burn, or **SB,** is the actual flame, the consumption of those food "logs." In scientific terms, **SB** is calculated by dividing the amount of carbon dioxide you exhale (a waste product of metabolism) by the amount of oxygen you consume (vital for life-sustaining metabolism). The power of the fire you'll end up with depends on the composition of the food you eat.

Spark Fuel-Spark Burn Relationship

Spark Fuel CO_2/O_2	Percent of Calories From Carbohydrates	Percent of Calories From Fat	Spark Burn CO_2/O_2
1.00	100	0	1.00
0.95	83	17	0.95
0.90	67	33	0.90
0.85	50	50	0.85
0.80	33	67	0.80
0.75	17	83	0.75
0.70	0	100	0.70

Most people fall somewhere in the middle, eating foods that are a balance of fats and carbs and burning carbs and fats fairly equally. Their weight stays pretty much in the same range.

If you have a low **SB,** your body is burning more fat—*which gives you the optimal metabolic upper hand.*

If you have a high **SB,** your body is burning less fat and it's not going near the stored stuff. You will be gaining—not losing fat. In other words, you'll be putting on the pounds.

In short:

- If your **SF** and **SB** are equal, you will maintain your weight.
- If your **SF** is consistently greater than your **SB,** you will lose weight.
- If your **SF** is consistently lower than your **SB,** you will gain weight.

What does all this have to do with the Spark? Plenty. Obviously, if you want to lose weight, you'll want to maintain a **higher SF–lower SB** relationship. You'll want to get that fire to "spark" on the first take.

And the best way to get and maintain a weight-loss "spark" is to:

1. ***Lower your SB with exercise.*** In fact, the Spark workouts, a combination of aerobic and strength-training quick bursts, are the most effective way to lower your **SB** fast. By enhancing the release of fat-mobilizing hormones (GH, adrenaline, and nor-adrenaline) and fat oxidation, the Spark exercises are designed to keep your **SB** low *even after you've stopped.* This translates into even more stored fat getting burned hour after hour.
2. ***Raise your SF with a diet high in fiber.*** Your muscles crave high-fiber carbs. And the fiber-rich complex carbohydrates recommended on the Spark Food Plan are the ideal route to high **SF.** *Counting fiber—not calories—optimizes your ability to burn the excess body fat accumulated over years* of inactivity and a diet too rich in fats and too low in fiber.

Sound complicated? Not to worry. The Spark plan already has the **SF-SB** equation built into it. I've done the work for you and the people in the Spark study have performed the hands-on test—successfully. With only *slight* adjustments in diet, an additional fruit and vegetable during the day, a pass on butter and creamy salad dressings at lunch, and the right combination of exercise Sparks, each participant had a weight loss that was *right for him or her,* a healthy weight loss that averaged 3 pounds within the first three weeks.

As these facts demonstrate, the two components of the Spark plan (exercise Sparks and food Sparks) will minimize the number of calories stored as fat. Your muscles will be soaking up the carbs you eat; the more exercise you do, the more your muscles will soak them up. Not only will your muscles be too busy to store calories, but they'll be burning up whatever you happen to have on the shelves. Fat anyone?

Together, the Spark exercise and food plans will keep you satisfied faster and longer; you'll want to eat less fat—*which means you'll have less fat to burn.* Your equation will be at the ideal place for losing weight and keeping it off: high **SF,** low **SB.**

This is, to quote the vernacular, "a good thing"—but it is *particularly* good for people over fifty. As we age, we lose our capacity to burn fat after a calorie-laden meal. This means that a great many of those calories are stored as fat and we'll gain weight—if we don't keep our **SF** high and our **SB** low.

But there is hope, and its name is exercise. As I have proved in the Spark study and other research I've conducted over the years, a single bout of exercise, especially when fueled by carbs, stimulates fat burning after exercise. Make that Spark-like exercise, strategically timed, and you will not only minimize fat storage after a meal, but you will actually accelerate the fat-burning process!

SPARKLER

"I lost 3 pounds just doing 15 Sparks a week and eating like I normally do. And I can tell they're the kind of pounds that will stay off."

—MARY W., a participant in the Spark Study 2000

SPARK ATTACKS

You've now seen the evidence. You've seen how the Spark Study 2000 at the University of Virginia exploded all the preconceptions we have about exercise, diet, and metabolism.

But there's still that small voice, the skeptic that has believed the diet myths for too long to just let them go. For those of you out there like Joanne H., Dianne V., and the other thirty-eight participants in the Spark study who simply couldn't believe that three weeks could make such a difference, the next few pages should help you finally let go of your preconceptions and miscalculations of diet and exercise. I call my explanations of these fitness myths Spark Attacks because they get right to the point, clean, fast, and irrefutably the last word.

SPARK ATTACK # 1: The More You Work Out, the More Body Fat You'll Burn

You can walk from today till a month of Sundays, but if your goal is to burn fat, you'll literally be on a treadmill. One of the most popular beliefs in the fitness world over the past twenty years is that in order to effectively burn fat you need to exercise for a long duration within the so-called fat-burning zone. This zone, a notch below the cardiovascular fitness zone on your gym's heart rate chart or aerobic machine's display, is where many instructors feel you need to be—for at least 30 to 40 minutes per session—in order to lose body fat.

This rationale actually stems from two myths:

1. You don't even start burning fat until some 20 or 30 minutes after you start to exercise.
2. Low-intensity exercise is best for burning fat.

Wrong. You start burning fat during the *first minute* of exercise . . . and keep on burning fat even after you stop. This has been demonstrated time and again in published reports from exercise physiology labs around the world.

However, it is true that at a lower exercise intensity, fat comprises a greater *percentage* of total calories burned. *But this misses the whole picture.* Higher-intensity exercise actually burns more fat calories. For example, even though at first glance 90 percent of 5 calories burned per minute during a long, less intensive workout sounds like a lot, *it is still less than 60 percent of 10 calories burned per minute during shorter but high-intensity Spark-like bouts done 7–10 times a week.*

In other words, there really is no such thing as a "fat-burning zone."

Need more convincing? The "afterburn" you get after exercise, that metabolism boost, is much stronger after a high-intensity workout. Since you're burning fewer calories in a fat-burning zone, your metabolism isn't stimulated as much afterward.

And here's another plus: The more carbohydrates you burn during exercise, the more fat you will burn *after* exercise. Any carbs you eat after exercise will be preferentially directed straight to carbohydrate-depleted muscles and the liver (which have burned up their carb supply during the bout of vigorous exercise you just did). Since muscles and the liver depend on carbohydrates to function, your body makes sure these organs get refueled first. Translation? Since the carbs you eat are being stored for the muscles and the liver, they aren't converted to fat—*which means your body must burn its own fat.* Instead of thinking of exercise as a fat-burning tool, think of it as a carbohydrate-burning—and even fun—way to lose excess fat.

The exercise Sparks are structured to create this metabolic advantage: short enough (10 minutes!) to be able to go at optimal intensity and frequent enough to take advantage of *multiple* afterburns. A much better use of your time and your body's fat-burning capabilities than a half-hour or so on the treadmill.

SPARK ATTACK # 2: Beware the High Glycemic

The glycemic index is a measure of how high your blood sugar goes up after you consume various carbohydrates. Some carbs are labeled high glycemic because they cause your blood sugar to rise more than others; the acutely elevated blood sugar causes more insulin to be secreted. Since insulin is a hormone that facilitates fat storage, the popular low-carb diet books lay out the scenario that high glycemic index foods cause (1) a blood sugar rush, which (2) causes a surge in insulin, which, in turn, (3) causes you to store the carbs as fat.

Wrong. To rank foods solely on the basis of glycemic index is overly simplistic. Although the glycemic index is based on sound science, classifying carbs as "good" or "bad" based solely on their glycemic index is not. *All* carbohydrates have nutritional value and can be a part of a healthful diet. For example, carrots, potatoes, watermelon, whole wheat bread, Cheerios, and corn flakes all have a high glycemic index. These foods certainly aren't "bad" or fattening.

The people who participated in the Spark study all ate a high-carbohydrate, low-fat diet. I asked them to simply add more complex carbs to their diet (with no differentiation between high and low glycemic foods) and reduce the amount of fat they consumed without counting calories. *At the end of the third week, 90 percent of the participants had lost weight.*

SPARK ATTACK # 3: Go That Extra Mile When You're Fitness Walking! More Effort Means a Bigger Return

Conventional wisdom on fitness walking, summed up from the many studies on the subject, suggests that:

1. Fitness benefits and weight loss are best realized when you burn at least 1,000 calories per week (which for most people translates to about 12 to 13 miles for that week)—a big commitment and a lot of walking!
2. Aerobic fitness can be expected to increase by 10 to 20 percent within a few months.

The Spark changes all this.

Women and men in the Spark program averaged between eight and nine 10-minute aerobic Sparks per week—or only about 400 calories per week and only 4 to 5 miles' worth of walking. And yet their improvement in aerobic fitness was about 15 percent—the same as reported in the 12- to 13-mile-per-week studies. The people in the conventional studies did their fitness walking in bouts of 30 to 60 minutes, four to five times a week. The Spark study participants simply grabbed 10-minute aerobic intervals eight to nine times during the week.

Conventions are about to change. The Spark Study 2000 is proving it with every participant:

"Thanks for the opportunity to participate in a program that produced so much gain for so little input," said Ancil C., a fifty-six-year-old corporate executive.

"Short exercise segments," said Mary W., *"proved to me that less can be more."*

Spark Attack # 4: You'll Live Longer If You're Thin

We might be programmed to spurn obesity in ourselves and others, but as I wrote in my 1996 book, *Big Fat Lies: The Truth About Your Weight and Your Health,* it is not being fat that hurts us, it's not being fit.

For overweight people who are in good health and reasonably fit, there is no compelling evidence to link lowered mortality rates with weight loss. It just doesn't exist. Rather, obesity might be an indicator of other risk factors, such as poor diet and sedentary lifestyle.

In fact, exercise is the great equalizer. If you are fat and you exercise regularly, you are as well off healthwise as your thinner counterparts who also exercise. A 1999 study of 21,925 men conducted by Dr. Steven Blair and his colleagues at the Cooper Institute for Aerobics Research in Dallas, and reported in the *American Journal of Clinical Nutrition,* supports this claim. In this study, men who were fat but fit had death rates equal to men who were lean and fit. Indeed, they had *half* the death rate of their thin, but unfit, counterparts. Data from this study also showed that low fitness in fat men was as strong or stronger a predictor of mortality as diabetes, high cholesterol, high blood pressure, smoking, or actually having cardiovascular disease itself.

In short, fitness is the great equalizer—and predictor of longevity. Body weight, body fat, and waist size have nothing to do with mortality as long as you are fit. The good news is that my Spark Study 2000 showed an improvement in aerobic capacity equivalent to the fitness level of *someone ten to fifteen years younger. This translates into a drop in mortality rates by at least 25 percent—in only three weeks!*

Metabolic fitness, the phrase I made popular in *Big Fat Lies,* is a much better indicator of health and well-being than your weight—in pounds or body fat. Your metabolism is the sum of all the chemical processes, both good and bad, that go on in your body. Broadly speaking, being metabolically fit means having a metabolism that maximizes

---

SPARK PLUG

Two separate studies published in the *New England Journal of Medicine,* one in 1991 and another in 1998, reported that aerobic exercise, coupled with a low-fat diet, could reduce cholesterol levels in women by 11 to 17 mg/dl in 9 to 12 months.

The women participating in the Spark study achieved a reduction in cholesterol that averaged 15 mg/dl—in 3 weeks.

Some exciting implications: a 1 percent reduction in cholesterol is thought to reduce coronary heart disease risk by 3 percent. The Spark Study 2000 women dropped their average cholesterol from 218 to 203—or a 7 percent reduction. **Certainly there are other things to consider with regard to health, but just using the cholesterol results alone, the women in the Spark study reduced their risk of coronary heart disease by 21 percent in only 3 weeks. The women in the two *New England Journal of Medicine* studies showed the same results—but after 9 to 12 months.**

---

vitality and minimizes the risk of disease, particularly those diseases that are influenced by lifestyle, such as heart disease, adult-onset diabetes, and cancer. It can be achieved independent of body fat percentages and cardiovascular fitness; its benefits include improved cholesterol profiles, increased glucose tolerance (and less risk of high and low blood sugar swings), reduced insulin levels, lower blood pressure, and an enhanced capacity to remove fat from the bloodstream after meals. In fact, **a metabolically fit fifty-year-old has basically the same health risks as an average person twenty to thirty years younger.**

The Spark Study 2000 at the University of Virginia showed *immediate* results on blood glucose, cholesterol, and triglyceride levels.

SPARK ATTACK # 5: Sugar Makes You Fat

Guess again. Several studies report that sugar in the diet may be necessary for good weight control; there is no reason to suggest that eliminating sugar for the rest of your life is the route to weight control. Researchers at the University of Colorado Health Science Center in Denver reported in the *American Journal of Clinical Nutrition* that high intake of sugar is negatively associated with obesity. But high intake of fat is positively associated with obesity. In other words, it's not the sugar. Nor is it the carbs. Once again, it's the fat that makes you fat. That's why the Spark Food Plan has room for all foods, including sugar—and another reason why *100 percent* of the participants in the Spark study were able to stick to it!

K's Spark

I might be beautiful in my dreams, but I am never athletic. I've never crossed a finish line, hit a home run, or skated a perfect triple lutz. Being an athlete is so foreign to me that I couldn't even conjure up the image.

But, a long time ago, in junior high school, there was rock 'n' roll. It was the period after lunch and we were all in the gym and we were told we could dance. We could dance. I could dance. That was the one thing I could do, the one thing that didn't feel athletic, that didn't feel strenuous. It was free, rolling, smoking, jiving, the beat hitting the high wired windows and bouncing back to me. I could meet Jimmy, basketball hero and jock of my dreams, on my own terms. Dancing. Kicking my heels, twirling my arms, a perfect staccato to my friend Ellen. We were the fast and furious jitterbug queens at Woodrow Wilson Junior High.

I didn't think of myself as a dancer. I didn't think, Wow. I'm really hitting my target heart rate zone now. And I certainly didn't think of the ten-minute songs as Sparks.

I didn't think. I Sparked.

And it felt grand.

SPARKLER

"I've been walking my black Lab for five years now. I didn't know it, but I've been following the principle in the Spark. That's because I do it several times a day, rain or shine, no matter my mood. One day I noticed that I had increased my muscle tone, my lung capacity, and my energy. I have more energy now than I did in my twenties."

—FRAN P., a forty-five-year-old writer,
artist, and mother of two

CHAPTER 3

Making the Spark Work for You:
A Series of Self-Tests

> On March 13, 1986, Microsoft went public.
> Trading began at 9:35 A.M. at $25.75 a share. By
> the time the stock market closed later that day,
> Bill Gates had raised $61 million in his first
> offering—or about $2 million every 10 minutes.

K's Spark

I knew what stress tests were. Periodically, on the evening news, you'd see gray-haired people walking a treadmill, wired up to a machine. It looked effortless when you watched someone else do it. Even boring.

So when I was told I'd have to take one, I rose to the challenge. I'd just signed up for yet another weight-loss plan. This one was through a local hospital; it was geared to health, and exercise was encouraged. I didn't care what its philosophy was. It was new, different, and I was ready to give it a shot.

I entered the cardiovascular department where the test was

being conducted after I purposely ate what was for me a low-cal lunch (a BLT on light bread) and put on a new pair of stretch leggings (black).

A nurse set me up to the electrocardiogram then started the treadmill. The doctor came in and explained how the test worked. As I walked at a slight incline, the speed would get progressively faster. I was to go as long as I could, "stomp till you drop" kind of thing. As soon as I waved my arm or shouted "Stop!" the test would end. By pushing me to my aerobic limits, the test would be able to determine how efficiently oxygen pumped through my blood, which, ultimately, would determine how fit I was.

I smiled; I understood. The test began innocently enough. I walked; the electrocardiogram moved. The nurse nodded. The doctor checked my pulse. All was in order. I walked. The doctor stood on one side of me, the nurse on the other. I walked. Two minutes later, the pace picked up. Okay. I can still do this. The electrocardiogram moved faster. I walked. The doctor and the nurse began to discuss the movie *Wall Street,* which had just opened in a theater in town. The doctor liked it. The nurse didn't. I started to speak, "Yeah, it was good," but they had already begun talking about lunch. I walked. They talked. Favorite foods. The New Jersey Nets. The new hospital elevators. The cost of raising kids.

I started to slow. My breathing was slightly forced, but nothing urgent. I had just started to feel the strain; their conversation distracted me. I felt awful. I couldn't concentrate on my feet. I could tell that the doctor and the nurse didn't want to be there. In the middle of their conversation about Disney World, I held up my hand. "Stop."

The nurse took the tape and the wires off my torso. The doctor checked my heart, my pulse, and my eyes. Within thirty seconds, I was off the machine. They told me that I'd only gone about eight minutes. Less than average for a woman of my age and weight.

I wiped my face with a paper towel. I took a sip of water. I thanked the doctor and the nurse for their time. They left me, closing the door behind them. I felt like a failure.

I failed the test because I stopped. Not because I was out of breath, but because I felt I had been imposing on the doctor and his nurse.

I didn't blame them. There were simply doing their job. They weren't in that room to motivate me. That was my job.

Although it wasn't yet a word in my vocabulary, I "sparked" just then. I realized that motivation had to come from me and no one else. What I did with my life didn't really matter to anyone else (except D.J. and maybe my mom). I had to learn to put myself first because no one else would. And that was not only okay, but right.

Maybe I had passed the stress test after all.

I'm one of the lucky ones. Since I've always been athletic and healthy, I never needed to be tested for cardiovascular health. If one particular sport didn't suit me, there was another that did.

But in my capacity as an exercise physiologist and university professor, I've certainly given my share of tests. I also know that most of you need direction. You need to know where to start and how to make your workout work effectively for you.

In order to maximize the benefits that can come with the Spark program, to individualize it as much as possible for you and, most important to me, create a program that you'll stick to, I've devised a four-part series of self-tests, similar to the ones I used in the Spark Study 2000.

Part 1 will help you determine your own individual Spark equation, testing your level of fitness, strength, and flexibility so you'll know exactly how many aerobic, strength-training, and flexibility Sparks you need to do each week.

Part 2 looks at your health, to help you get the most out of your Spark. You'll find a simple body fat test and an exercise preparatory test.

Part 3 is all about food. You'll find a test to educate you on how to recognize real hunger and on appetite control, to help you recognize when and why you eat. You'll also take a short quiz on fiber and nutrition to ensure that, in the name of weight loss, you are not giving yourself *less* of a good thing.

Finally, in Part 4, you'll find the Spark "Style Section," a two-part test to help pinpoint your exercise preferences and your lifestyle choices; they are a kind of launchpad into the world of the Spark.

These tests, in various forms, have all been used by not only the participants in the Spark Study 2000, but by people who have heard about the Spark and started it on their own, people from all walks of life who desire, above all else, one thing: health. These tests have been designed to be fast, easy to do, and enlightening. You can do all eight at one time in less than an hour. You can do them alone or with a friend. And, except for the Spark fitness walk, which, unless you have a home treadmill, needs a high school track, a park, or a gym, they can all be done in the privacy of your own home. One hour. No fancy equipment. No complicated formulas. And once you've added up your answers, you'll not only be more enlightened about yourself, your mind, and your physical body, but you'll be ready to light *your* Spark.

PART 1: YOUR EXERCISE SPARK EQUATION

TEST 1: How Aerobically Fit Are You?
The Spark Fitness Walk Test

Aerobic fitness measures the strength of your heart and your lungs and it's a powerful predictor of overall health and risk of premature death. Data from the famed Cooper Institute indicates that low fitness is a major predicator of cardiovascular mortality. Simple improvements, such as the kind we saw in the Spark study, can greatly reduce mortality risk. To ensure that you start your aerobic Sparks with the appropriate amount of Sparks (not so high that you injure yourself or give up in frustration, not so low that you won't reap any benefits), take this short 1-mile walking test. Anyone can do it!

What you'll need:

- An indoor or outdoor track (most high schools and gyms have one), a home treadmill, or a flat, smooth block in the neighborhood.
- A digital watch (for easy viewing) or a stopwatch.
- Loose, easy clothing and comfortable walking shoes or sneakers.
- A reasonably empty stomach. Try not to eat for two hours before the test. (It might upset your stomach and slow you down.)

Doing the test:

1. Determine how many laps or blocks equal 1 mile, or use your home treadmill.
    ✔ Most school tracks are 4 laps per mile.

- ✔ A home treadmill will provide the information as you walk.

- ✔ For neighborhood walks, use your car odometer to determine how many blocks equal 1 mile.

  (For simplicity, the directions below will use outdoor track terminology.)

2. Walk slowly around the track for 2 to 3 minutes to warm up. Stretch.

3. Set your stopwatch (or note the time) and begin to walk briskly for 1 mile. Stay in the inside lane of the track. Try to maintain a constant pace and go as fast as you can without wearing yourself out.

4. Stop when you've finished your 1-mile walk. Jot down your time.

   The time you used to complete 1 mile:
   _____ minutes/_____ seconds

5. Continue to walk very slowly around the track for 2 to 3 minutes to cool down. This will allow your heart rate and blood pressure to return to normal.

6. Use the following charts to assess your aerobic fitness level. You'll need these results later to determine how many aerobic Sparks you'll be doing each week.

1-Mile Walk Scoring Table: Women

Fitness Category	Age 20–29	30–39	40–49	50–59	60+
Very High	≤12:30	≤13:00	≤13:30	≤14:00	≤15:00
High	12:31–14:00	13:01–14:30	13:31–15:00	14:01–15:30	15:01–16:30
Moderate	14:01–17:30	14:31–18:00	15:01–18:30	15:31–19:00	16:31–20:00
Low	>17:30	>18:00	>18:30	>19:00	>20:00

1-Mile Walk Scoring Table: Men

Fitness Category	Age 20–29	30–39	40–49	50–59	60+
Very High	≤12:00	≤12:30	≤13:00	≤13:30	≤14:30
High	12:01–13:30	12:31–14:00	13:01–14:30	13:31–15:00	14:31–16:00
Moderate	13:31–17:00	14:01–17:30	14:31–18:00	15:01–18:30	16:01–19:30
Low	>17:00	>17:30	>18:00	>18:30	>19:30

Check one: My aerobic fitness category is

☐ **Low**
☐ **Moderate**
☐ **High**
☐ **Very High**

If it took you longer to walk the mile than you had hoped, do not feel discouraged. These tests are not designed to prepare you for competition. Nor are they a competition in and of themselves. Your answers are used to determine the Spark plan best for you, nothing more and nothing less. The Spark works equally well for those who "feel the

---

SPARKLER

"I wanted to get going on some kind of program. That was my goal. I ended up doing 11 or 12 aerobic Sparks a week, which improved my 1-mile walk time by 2 minutes and 15 seconds. I not only reached my goal, but I'm still going strong. Without taking one or two hours out of my day like most exercise programs."

—PAT S., forty-three, real estate broker, mother of two, and initial Spark study participant

---

burn" during a stroll in the park as it does for those of you who can easily do an Alpine hike.

The women in the Spark Study 2000 (with an average age of forty-five) did their 1-mile self-test in 16 minutes, 50 seconds, which put them at the Moderate level. After three weeks, they redid the test and improved their time by over 1 minute—reducing their 1-mile walk time to 15 minutes, 45 seconds and going strong!

TEST 2: How Strong Are Your Muscles? The Spark Strength Test

Muscular strength is a key to a good quality of life. It provides a sense of well-being, energy, and overall physical health. But another fact of life is that we lose a significant amount of muscle mass as we age, particularly after the age of fifty. By doing the strength-training exercises in the Spark plan, you'll help reduce age-related muscle loss—and improve bone health, which is crucial for postmenopausal women. If you increase your strength now, you'll reduce your risk of falls and injury later.

To know how many strength-training Sparks you'll need, take these two easy tests. They will measure your muscular fitness, as well as your upper-body and abdominal muscular endurance.

Push-Up Test for the Upper Body (Deltoids, Pectorals, and Triceps)

What you'll need:

- A stopwatch, a digital watch, or a watch with a second hand. You'll need to gauge a minute.
- A sponge block or rolled-up towel or blanket.

- A carpeted floor or an exercise mat to support your knees.
- Loose, comfortable clothing.

Doing the test:

For women:

1. Start with a few light stretches, rolling your shoulders and moving your head from side to side, to limber yourself up.
2. Kneel down on the floor. Place your hands about shoulder-width apart; arms should be fully extended and fingers spread and pointed forward.
3. Put the block or rolled-up blanket or towel on the floor under your chest. It should be about 3 to 4 inches thick.
4. The push-up begins in this up position: Knees are on the floor, but your weight is supported by your arms and palms. Your back and upper legs are in a straight line.

5. Bend your arms at the elbow to lower your chest until it reaches the block or towel.
6. Push yourself back up to the starting position: arms straight, palms facing down, fingers spread and straight out. (It's okay if your feet come up off the floor during the push-up.)
7. Bring your body back down to the towel, then push yourself up. Inhale on the way down; exhale on the way up.
8. Repeat the push-up. Do as many as you can for 1 minute.
   I completed _____ push-ups.
9. Assess your level of upper-body strength with the following charts, adapted from the Cooper Institute for Aerobics Research, Dallas, Texas.

For men:

1. Do this same push-up, but with your feet extended behind you and your knees lifted up. Your weight will be supported by your palms and your toes; your body should be in a straight line from your back to your legs.
2. Repeat the push-up. Do as many as you can for 1 minute.
   I completed _____ push-ups.
3. Assess your level of upper body strength with the following charts.

Push-Up Scoring Table: Women (Modified Push-Up)

			Age		
Fitness Category	**20–29**	**30–39**	**40–49**	**50–59**	**60+**
Very High	≥36	≥31	≥24	≥21	≥15
High	30–35	24–30	18–23	17–20	12–14
Moderate	8–29	12–23	7–17	7–16	3–11
Low	≤7	≤11	≤6	≤6	≤2

Push-Up Scoring Table: Men (Full Push-Up)

Fitness Category	20–29	30–39	Age 40–49	50–59	60+
Very High	≥47	≥39	≥30	≥25	≥23
High	37–46	30–38	24–29	19–24	18–22
Moderate	23–36	18–29	12–23	10–18	7–17
Low	≤22	≤17	≤11	≤9	≤6

Check one: My upper-body muscular fitness is

☐ **Low**
☐ **Moderate**
☐ **High**
☐ **Very High**

The average number of push-ups the women who participated in the Spark Study 2000 did on their first self-test go-around was an average of 10 in 1 minute. This made sense, since the majority of the participants did no strength-training exercise prior to the study. (Upper body strength is notoriously low in middle-aged women in general.)

But after 3 weeks on the Spark plan, the average number of push-ups these women did in 1 minute was 22! They went from a moder-

---

SPARKLER

"The Spark also makes a great postpartum exercise program. It's not too strenuous. You can walk a little, lift weights, and stretch some right after you've had a baby without risk. And 10-minute increments are enough to give you a lift throughout the day."

—MARY W., participant in the Spark Study 2000
and mother of three

---

ately fit level to a highly fit level. In other words, *they jumped beyond 45 percent of their peer population in just 3 weeks and had the muscular endurance equivalent to women 10 to 15 years younger.*

Sit-Up Test for Your Abdominals

What you'll need:

- Exercise mat or carpeted floor
- A nearby bed or piece of furniture with a small space between the floor and the bottom (to anchor your feet) or a friend to hold your feet down
- Digital watch, stopwatch, or watch with a second hand (to time 1 minute)
- Loose, comfortable clothing

Doing the test:

1. Warm up by marching in place 1 or 2 minutes.
2. Lie back on your mat, your knees bent, your legs together. Feet should be flat on the floor. (The mat should be near the bed, so your feet are anchored beneath it. Or, better yet, have someone hold your feet down.)
3. Cross your arms in front of your chest.
4. Slowly sit up, using your stomach muscles—*not your neck*—to pull you up as far as you can go.

     ✔ *A word of caution: If you have any back problems, I suggest skipping this test. If you are starting out feeling very weak, do crunches instead, curling up just until your shoulder blades lift off the floor. You can progress to full sit-ups during your strength-training Sparks as you get stronger.*

5. Move back down until your shoulders just touch the mat.
6. Repeat. Do as many as you can in 1 minute. Try to breathe as normally as you can, exhaling as you come up, inhaling as you go down.

   Number of sit-ups in 1 minute: _____
7. Use the charts below to assess your level of abdominal strength, adapted from the Cooper Institute for Aerobics Research, Dallas, Texas.

Sit-Up Scoring Table: Women

Fitness Category	20–29	30–39	Age 40–49	50–59	60+
Very High	≥44	≥35	≥29	≥24	≥17
High	38–43	29–34	24–28	20–23	11–16
Moderate	25–37	21–28	15–23	11–19	4–10
Low	≤24	≤20	≤14	≤10	≤3

Sit-Up Scoring Table: Men

Fitness Category	20–29	30–39	Age 40–49	50–59	60+
Very High	≥47	≥45	≥39	≥35	≥30
High	42–46	39–44	34–38	28–34	22–29
Moderate	34–41	31–38	25–33	20–27	16–21
Low	≤33	≤30	≤24	≤19	≤15

Check one: My abdominal muscular fitness is

- ☐ **Low**
- ☐ **Moderate**
- ☐ **High**
- ☐ **Very High**

Maybe you can't do more than one or two sit-ups right now, but improvement is on the way—most likely within three (Spark) weeks. The average improvement for participants in the Spark study was 50 percent, up from 14 sit-ups during the initial self-test to 21 after they'd been on the Spark for three weeks. Joanne H., a fifty-year-old associate professor and mother of two college-aged kids, increased the number of sit-ups she did by 85 percent, jumping from 20 in the first self-test to 37 after three weeks. She's not alone. Many of the participants jumped two whole fitness categories, from Low to High; from Moderate to Very High—*the equivalent fitness level of a person about fifteen years younger.*

Jot down your scores from the push-up test and the sit-up test. If both are Low, your average muscular strength score will be Low. Similarly, if both are Moderate, your score will be Moderate; and if both are High, your score will be High. If one is Low and the other is High, consider your score as Moderate. However, if one test comes out Moderate and the other is either High or Low, still consider your muscular strength score as Moderate. This new average score for muscular strength will be used to determine how many strength-training Sparks you'll need to do each week.

Level for push-ups _____

Level for sit-ups _____

=

Average muscular strength: _____

TEST 3: How Flexible Are You? The Spark Stretch Test

Stress-relief might be the reason many people have taken up yoga in the past few years. But a not-so-inconsiderable side benefit is enhanced flexibility to your muscles and joints. With renewed flexibility, you can move with grace and vigor without fear of personal injury. You can enjoy a wider range of motion in your joints, bringing more pleasure to the activities you do. Even something as mundane as reaching for a can of soup on a high shelf or picking up your kid's clothing can be performed with less effort. Because flexibility is an important quality for a healthy life, my plan also figures in a variety of flexibility Sparks each week as part of your total. To determine where you'll start with your stretches, take this short test; it measures the flexibility of your lower back and the hamstring muscles in the back of your legs.

What you'll need:

- A 12-inch carton, box, bench, stepper, or even a stack of heavy books
- A yardstick (you'll find out why below)
- Loose, comfortable clothing (no shoes!)

Doing the test:

1. Tape the yardstick perpendicular to the top of the box, parallel to the floor; the 15-inch mark should be lined up with the edge of the box (see diagram).
2. Stretch out your arms and shake your legs to warm up.
3. Rest the bottoms of your stocking feet on the edge of the box; they should be right under the yardstick (which is in line with your legs and pointing right at your belly button).

4. With your hands together, arms straight out, lean forward slowly and reach as far as you can over the yardstick. Exhale. Hold this position for 2 seconds. Don't bounce or lunge. Keep your legs straight and on the floor.

5. Jot down the point on the yardstick where the tips of your middle fingers stretched to. Round the number to the nearest ½ inch. (Reaching to your toes would give you a score of 15.)

6. Repeat 2 more times, jotting down each answer. Use the highest number for your score.

   1st try: Farthest point I went was _____ inches.

   2nd try: Farthest point I went was _____ inches.

   3rd try: Farthest point I went was _____ inches.

   Highest score: _____ inches.

7. Use the charts below to determine your Spark flexibility category, adapted from the Cooper Institute for Aerobics Research, Dallas, Texas.

Flexibility Scoring Table: Women

Fitness Category	Age 20–29	30–39	40–49	50–59	60+
Very High	≥22.5	≥21.5	≥20.5	≥20.5	≥19.0
High	20.5–22.0	20.0–21.0	19.0–20.0	18.5–20.0	17.0–18.5
Moderate	17.5–20.0	17.0–19.5	15.5–18.5	15.5–18.0	13.5–16.5
Low	≤17.0	≤16.5	≤15.0	≤15.0	≤13.0

Flexibility Scoring Table: Men

Fitness Category	Age 20–29	30–39	40–49	50–59	60+
Very High	≥20.5	≥19.5	≥18.5	≥17.5	≥17.5
High	18.5–20.0	17.5–19.0	16.5–18.0	15.5–17.0	14.5–17.0
Moderate	15.0–18.0	13.5–17.0	12.5–16.0	11.0–15.0	10.5–14.0
Low	≤14.5	≤13.0	≤12.0	≤10.5	≤10.0

Check one: My flexibility is

☐ **Low**
☐ **Moderate**
☐ **High**
☐ **Very High**

Joanne H., a fifty-year-old participant in the Spark Study 2000, jumped from a Low level (9.5 inches) in her "sit-and-reach" flexibility self-test to a Moderate level at the end of three weeks—an improvement of 6.5 inches. *Her ability to stretch is now equivalent to a thirty-year-old's!* She is not alone. The average improvement for all the participants in the flexibility category was 2.6 inches in three weeks.

This ends the "physically active" part of the Spark self-tests. It's time to see what you've got. Jot down the scores from each of the three previous tests below:

Scores:

1. **The Spark Aerobic Fitness Test** _____
2. **The Spark Muscular Strength Test** _____
3. **The Spark Flexibility Stretch Test** _____

To create your exercise Spark equation, find your scores in the following models (*Note: These equations are to be used as guides only. From my years of research as well as from the results of my Spark study at the University of Virginia, I suggest trying to make the most of your aerobic Sparks by doing from 7 to 10 each week, with the balance mixed between strength and flexibility.*)

For Aerobic Sparks:

If you scored:	Try this many per week:
Low	9 to 10
Moderate	8
High or Very High	7

For Strength-Training Sparks:

If you scored:	Try this many per week:
Low	4
Moderate	3
High or Very High	2

For Flexibility Sparks:

If you scored:	Try this many per week:
Low	4
Moderate	3
High or Very High	2

If you scored Low in all three tests, use this equation:

9 aerobic Sparks

3 strength-training Sparks

3 flexibility Sparks

After three weeks, redo your self-tests and (since I'm sure you'll see an improvement!) change your equation accordingly, using the standard exercise models.

Here's an example to help you create your Spark equation, using Joanne H., our "poster child" for the Spark because she saw so much improvement in every area during her three weeks:

Joanne's initial test indicated

Moderate, for aerobic Sparks

Moderate, for strength-training Sparks

Low, for flexibility Sparks

According to the models, her plan for the 3 weeks was

8 aerobic Sparks

3 strength-training Sparks

4 flexibility Sparks

. . . for a total of 15 10-minute Sparks a week.

Here's another example, using Dianne V., the thirty-eight-year-old college student, as an example:

Dianne's initial tests indicated

Low, for aerobic Sparks

Low, for strength-training Sparks

Moderate, for flexibility Sparks

SPARKLER

"I am forty-eight years old and I wanted to get to the point in my life where exercise is a part of my life . . . and now it is. And that's significant for me. The first three weeks really made a difference."

—DARCI L., full-time mom of two grade-school children and Spark Study participant

---

According to the models, her plan for the 3 weeks was

8 aerobic Sparks
4 strength-training Sparks
3 flexibility Sparks

. . . for a total of 15 10-minute Sparks a week.

The next part of your self-tests looks at your body, in particular your body fat and your health. As with the physical tests, the answers are meant to inform, only that. I will not judge you—and I hope that you won't judge yourself.

PART 2: A BRIEF LOOK AT YOUR HEALTH

TEST 4: How Much "Bad" Body Fat Do You Have? The Spark Waist Measurement Test

Body fat, understandably, has a bad name. It is the *look* of obesity, the fat you can't hide from the outside world, no matter how many dark-colored layers you pile on. Nevertheless, body fat, however it might appear to the naked eye, serves a definite purpose; the layer of subcutaneous fat right beneath the skin stores food, keeps you warm, and helps absorb bumps, bruises, knocks, and falls. Numerous studies, both in the United States and in Canada, have also found considerable evidence that subcutaneous fat around your thighs, the fat you "love to hate," may actually lower your risk of heart disease. The "pear shape" so hated by millions of women may actually be the shape of a healthy heart.

But there is "bad" body fat that is less obvious to the naked eye. This body fat, most of which is located deep within the abdominal area, around your internal organs, is called intra-abdominal, or visceral, fat. Too much of this visceral fat and your belly will swell, causing the "apple shape" seen more on men than women. (Although protruding bellies can be a result of too much subcutaneous fat, more times than not it is the deep visceral variety.) This visceral fat tends to be metabolically hyperactive, taking in, storing, and releasing fat into the bloodstream at breakneck speed. Unfortunately, this broken-down fat is in the form of free fatty acids, which can increase your risk of heart rhythm irregularities and impair your liver function to the degree that you become insulin resistant or diabetic. Visceral fat has also been associated with high cholesterol, high blood pressure, and high triglyceride levels.

In other words, *total percentage of body fat is less an indicator of health than location.*

The simple test I've devised below will help you estimate whether you have a level of intra-abdominal or "bad" body fat that may put you at high risk for health problems. The Spark plan will help everyone, regardless of your shape, but having an estimate of the amount of "bad" body fat you have will help you calculate where to start your Spark and what types of Sparks you should do.

What you'll need:

- A tape measure
- A pencil to jot down your answers below

Doing the test:

1. Measure your waist while standing in a relaxed stance. No sucking in your stomach! This measurement should reflect the largest circumference around your belly. (Typically, this is at the level of your navel. If you have a substantial amount of fat around your midsection, the largest circumference might be slightly above.)

   Waist circumference: _____ inches

2. Find your results on the following charts. This will give you a good idea of how much "bad" body fat you have.

Waist Circumference and Health Risk: Women Under 40 Years of Age

Low Risk ⟵———————⟶ Moderate Risk ⟵———————⟶ High Risk

| <26 | 27 | 28 | 29 | 30 | 31 | 32 | 33 | 34 | 35 | 36 | 37 | 38 | 39 | 40+ |

Waist Circumference (Inches)

Waist Circumference and Health Risk: Women Age 40 and Older

Low Risk ⟵———————⟶ Moderate Risk ⟵———————⟶ High Risk

| <26 | 27 | 28 | 29 | 30 | 31 | 32 | 33 | 34 | 35+ |

Waist Circumference (Inches)

Waist Circumference and Health Risk: Men Under 40 Years of Age

Low Risk ←—————→ Moderate Risk ←—————→ High Risk

<31	32	33	34	35	36	37	38	39	40+

Waist Circumference (Inches)

Waist Circumference and Health Risk: Men Age 40 and Older

Low Risk ←—————→ Moderate Risk ←—————→ High Risk

<31	32	33	34	35+

Waist Circumference (Inches)

Check one: My body fat puts me at

☐ **High Risk**
☐ **Moderate Risk**
☐ **Low Risk**

Low Risk does not mean "no risk," and High Risk does not mean that you should be buying a burial plot! Where you find yourself on these charts tells you nothing about your lifestyle, which must be considered before coming to any final conclusions about your risks. Getting fit, becoming active, eating a high-fiber diet—all these can change your risk. And all these variables will begin to do their "magic" the very first day you start your Spark. *Within three weeks of doing the Spark, your health risks will drop considerably—as they did for every single person who participated in the Spark Study 2000.*

> *Question: I realize that triglyceride levels are important,*
> *but they feel so abstract. What are they exactly—and when*
> *am I at risk?*
>
> *Answer:* Although their name might sound like they deal with
> higher math, triglycerides are a blood fat also found abundantly
> in—surprise!—fat cells. High numbers have been associated
> with the risk of heart disease. Numbers over 200 are considered
> borderline-high. Numbers from 400 to 1,000 are considered
> high. And anything over 1,000 is considered very high. Optimal
> triglyceride levels are anything under 110. *The majority of*
> *the participants in the Spark study reduced their triglyceride*
> *levels to the* **athletic** *range (the level of highly fit individuals)*
> *within the three-week period. Joanne H. reduced hers from 127*
> *to 101!*

Test 5: How Far Can You Spark?

Starting any new exercise or diet regimen is, on some level, un-
charted territory. You might know the basics. You might understand
the chemistry. But you need to make sure you are *capable* of the program you are about to start. This test provides some questions you
need to ask yourself before you begin.

Adapted from the Canadian Society for Exercise Physiology test
that is used worldwide, these seven easy questions will help you pinpoint any medical conditions that might influence how you begin the
Spark.

Answer yes or no to the following:

Yes	No	
☐	☐	1. Have you ever been diagnosed with a heart condition that could curtail your physical activities?
☐	☐	2. Have you ever felt pain in your chest when doing any physical activity, from shoveling snow and raking leaves to carrying groceries into the house?
☐	☐	3. In the past few weeks have you felt any chest pains when you were doing nothing more than lying on the couch?
☐	☐	4. Have you ever felt so dizzy that you've lost your balance?
☐	☐	5. Have you been diagnosed with any joint, bone, or muscle condition that could inhibit your ability to exercise?
☐	☐	6. Are you taking blood pressure medication or any other medications for your heart?
☐	☐	7. Are there any other medical reasons why you are cautious about beginning the Spark?

Total yes answers: _____
Total no answers: _____

The Spark plan can improve your quality of life—and reduce your risk of heart disease. But the Spark self-tests can only offer an indication of where you are right now. Obviously, they cannot take the place of a blood test in your doctor's office if:

- You find that the results of your self-tests are consistently low
- You've answered yes to *any* of the questions in the *How Far Can You Spark* self-test
- Your answers to the *How Much "Bad" Body Fat Do You Have* self-test put you in a high-risk category

In such cases, I strongly suggest you make an appointment with your doctor before starting this program. He or she can ensure your safety as well as prescribe medication that will only enhance the Spark's fire.

And here's the good news: For the people in the Spark study, the biggest improvements were observed in those who had the highest risks to begin with. In other words, the worse shape you are in when you start the Spark, the better the plan works for you!

Now it's on to Part 3, the group of self-tests that deal with one of my family's favorite subjects: food.

PART 3: FOOD FOR THOUGHT

TEST 6: How Much Do You Know about the Foods You Eat? The "Spark Your Food IQ" Fiber and Cholesterol Test

Fiber-rich carbohydrates are at the core of the Spark Food Plan. Thanks to the high **Spark Fuel**–low **Spark Burn** relationship built into the program, your body will be burning accumulated excess body fat. You'll feel fuller faster and longer. And, with muscles blazing from exercise and hearty fiber-rich complex carbohydrates, you'll go through your day with more energy and sleep better than you have in years.

By the end of three weeks on the Spark Food Plan, you'll be eating up to 25 grams of fiber a day—without doing anything more but making some better-informed choices. To get you thinking in a "fiber-rich" way, take a few moments to answer the questions in this quiz. (Can you fathom that eating a bran muffin—with raisins—every day will help you lose weight and keep your **SF-SB** Spark equation fired up? High fiber wins out every time.)

Answer yes or no to the following questions:

Yes   No

☐ ☐ 1. I eat whole grain bread with my sandwiches.

☐ ☐ 2. I love fruit. I'll eat two or three servings a day, an apple here, a pear there, a tangerine in the middle of the afternoon.

☐ ☐ 3. I'll take a plate of pasta marinara over a steak anytime.

☐ ☐ 4. I try to eat a salad at lunch or dinner—or both.

☐ ☐ 5. I order brown rice instead of white at the Chinese restaurant.

☐ ☐ 6. I eat breakfast every day, usually some toast and low-fat cheese or cereal and milk.

☐ ☐ 7. I nibble between meals. There's always food— veggies, fruit, rice cakes, or crackers—at my desk.

☐ ☐ 8. I avoid creamy dressings, preferring to drizzle olive oil and balsamic vinegar on my greens. I'll add some nuts and some dried fruits for texture.

☐ ☐ 9. I eat red meat rarely, perhaps a hamburger or a steak once a month. Instead, I'll opt for beans.

☐ ☐ 10. I love pretzels.

☐ ☐ 11. Bring on the desserts, the richest, the gooiest, and the most chocolatey—just not every single day. Most nights, I'll have fruit for dessert.

☐ ☐ 12. Thanks to salsa, I'll munch on celery and carrots all afternoon.

☐ ☐ 13. I get creative with my yogurt. I'll add strawberries, wheat germ, granola, even nuts. By the time I'm done, it's lunch.

☐ ☐ 14. I look for the word *bran* in my breakfast cereal.

Write down the number of yes-column answers you had for these questions. This is your Fiber Factor. The higher the number, the better the carbohydrate-rich fiber you already eat—and the easier you'll be able to Spark.

Fiber Factor: _____

No matter how much improvement you might feel your diet needs after taking this test, the Spark will be there, helping your body bring these factors into balance, ensuring a system that breaks down, stores, and burns food (fuel) efficiently. The result? Good health—and a slimmer body to boot.

Question: Why is cholesterol a predictor of heart disease?

Answer: Cholesterol is a waxy substance naturally made by your body. Everyone has some cholesterol in his or her bloodstream. It's not the cholesterol per se that puts you at risk of heart disease, it's the amount *and type.*

"Bad" LDL (low-density lipoprotein) cholesterol is the worst culprit. This waxy substance clings to artery walls as blood streams through our systems. The more buildup, the less efficiently our blood can pass through. LDL is affected most by saturated fat in your diet. LDL, or "bad" cholesterol, numbers between 130 and 159 are considered borderline high and should be checked regularly. Numbers over 160 are considered high risk and need a doctor's supervision. Anything under 130 is considered desirable. *On average, participants in the Spark study dropped from the borderline-high risk category to the desirable range.*

(continued)

On the other hand, you want more "good" HDL (high-density lipoprotein) cholesterol. This type acts like a "rotor-rooter," cleaning the LDL off the artery walls. The more HDL you have in your bloodstream, the "cleaner" your artery walls. Anything under 35 is considered high risk; over 60 is desirable.

An important indicator of cardiovascular disease risk is the ratio of the "bad" LDL cholesterol to the "good" HDL. Ratios below 3.0 are considered optimal, and anything above 5.0 is considered high risk. The average of the participants of the Spark Study 2000 was 4.5, not bad—but not great, either. But, within the study's 3 weeks, the average improvement was just under 0.4—or nearly 10 percent. And, *for the handful of people who had initial ratios above 5.0, the average drop was closer to 1.0— and each 1.0-unit drop corresponds to a 53 percent drop in cardiovascular disease risk.*

Test 7: Am I Hungry Yet?
The Spark Appetite Satiation Test

Inactivity is only one of the reasons people gain weight. Studies also show that you can pile on the extra pounds because you eat when you are not truly hungry—and you don't stop when you are full. This phenomenon has been described as a "dieting mentality," a state of mind in which people end up ignoring their bodies' internal cues of satiety and hunger and instead let an external diet do the decision making for them. They'll try to lose weight based on someone else's idea of portion control, body size, and taste. But external means are doomed to fail; you need to individualize a diet plan and make it work for you. People who have been the most successful in losing weight and keeping it off did not follow diets blindly. Instead, they incorporated the insights they gained about food and activity into their lifestyles.

The Spark Food Plan is based on the idea that you are an adult, that you can make decisions for yourself, that you can control your weight. And the first step toward that control is recognizing the cues that make you turn to food. Some of them are emotional, some of them are based on habit, some of them are based on an ingrained idea of self-deprivation, and some of them are based on very real appetite.

Take a few moments to complete the following self-test and see if you eat according to your stomach. This *Spark Your Appetite Scale* was adapted from one devised by registered dietitians Karin Kratina, Nancy King, and Dayle Hayes. Rate how each food situation makes you feel, from 1 to 5.

SPARK YOUR APPETITE SCALE

1. You're starving and everything on the menu looks good.
2. You're hungry and notice it's time for lunch.
3. You're neutral. You could eat, but you can also wait awhile.
4. Satisfyingly full. What a great meal!
5. Stuffed. Your waistband hurts.

Rating   ***Common Food Situations***

____   1. It's lunchtime at the office.

____   2. You're late for work and you rush out the door without breakfast.

____   3. You're getting ready to go to the newest hot spot for dinner.

(continued)

SPARK YOUR APPETITE SCALE *(cont.)*

Rating	Common Food Situations
____	4. It's evening and the TV is on—your cue to eat.
____	5. You don't order dessert and watch everyone else eat theirs.
____	6. You order dessert and eat every morsel.
____	7. You're driving in your car and thinking about stopping at a fast-food exit.
____	8. It's another night in a strange city, you're exhausted from your business trip, and you're not sure about ordering a room-service dinner.
____	9. You're reading a book in bed before you go to sleep and thinking about going to the kitchen for a snack.
____	10. You finished a meal about an hour ago and you pass a pastry shop.
____	11. The movie is going to start in five minutes.
____	12. You're at a business lunch.
____	13. It's three o'clock: the candy hour at the office.
____	14. You're on vacation.
____	15. You weigh yourself every day, sometimes twice.

There are no right or wrong answers to this test. It is devised to give you "food for thought," an awareness of when you eat and why.

If you consistently answered a 4, eating when you are satiated, or a 5, eating when you are stuffed, you need to pause before you pick up the fork, to distract yourself. (A 10-minute Spark is ideal, if possible!) Try to de-stress with relaxation strategies such as meditation, a flexibility Spark, or a plain and simple nap.

If you consistently answered a 1, eating when you are starving, you might be depriving yourself too much—which can lead to overeating when you eventually give yourself "permission" to eat.

The best balance is achieved when you consistently answer these questions with a 2, hungry, moving to a 3, neutral, or a 4, comfortably full. The Spark Food Plan helps you find this balance, offering a variety of high-fiber meals and snacks that promote satiety without "over the top" fullness—and encourages a "nibbling" eating style that avoids deprivation. The plan has already helped the participants in the Spark Study 2000 lose weight, drop clothing sizes, and feel more energetic. As Brenda M., a fifty-two-year-old office manager, says, *"By changing my eating habits, I am becoming aware of how much junk-type foods I was actually eating—mostly without even thinking about the food value."*

It's time to move on to the final portion of your Spark self-tests: your exercise style. These tests, too, will be used to personalize your Spark plan for results that work—and keep you motivated.

PART 4: THE SPARK STYLE SECTION

TEST 8: What Do You Want Out of Your Diet and Exercise Program? The Spark Launchpad Lifestyle Test

This last Spark self-test is, in some ways, the most important. By taking a moment to think about the following statements, you'll find a self-portrait emerging, a preference for diet and exercise that can mean the difference between a program that's doomed to fail and one you'll *want* to stay with for the rest of your life.

The first section of this test deals with your personality, the way you like to do things, the way you feel most comfortable. This will help you develop your own Spark program: either as a strict routine or more "free-flowing."

Answer true or false to the statements below:

Part 1: The Spark and My Personality

T F   1. I'm a high-energy individual. I don't like to sit still.

T F   2. I think things through. I consider myself a logical person.

T F   3. I'm a perfectionist.

T F   4. I hate my body.

T F   5. I hate to take naps.

T F   6. I wish I was easygoing and things rolled off my back. I'm fairly controlling.

T F   7. I try to read between the lines when it comes to people. The surface is only one part of the picture.

T F   8. I love routine.

T F   9. I keep organized schedules. I like to plan ahead.

T F   10. If someone needs something done, I'm the one to ask.

T F   11. I'm critical—of myself.

T F   12. I keep things close to my chest.

T F   13. I dislike showing my emotions.

T F   14. I dwell on the past.

You are probably aware of whether you are a flexible person or one who likes order. One is not better than the other, just different. Count the number of true statements and false statements you had.

Spark Personality Statements "true" total: _____

Spark Personality Statements "false" total: _____

The more "trues" you had, the more you'll need a structured exercise and food plan. The Spark provides organization, scheduling, and routine—if you need it.

If you had more "falses," you'll follow your own Spark, exercising and eating as the "spark hits." But the Spark program will still ensure that you get all your food and exercise Sparks in every week.

This next section briefly delves into your feelings about exercise itself. Do you like to move? Or are you hesitant to start?

PART 2: Exercise Your Passion

T F   1. Put music on and I'm ready to dance—but I won't.

T F   2. I *should* exercise.

T F   3. I only exercise when I diet. Quit the diet, and I quit exercising.

T F   4. If I miss a day or two of my diet or exercise regimen, I feel I've blown it and it's hard for me to get back on track.

T F   5. I feel intimidated by weight-resistance machines.

T F   6. I have a hard time keeping up with others in my aerobics classes.

T F   7. I don't feel water exercise is good enough—even though I love the water.

T F   8. I have a lot of aches and pains. I would never attempt yoga.

T F   9. My favorite activities are sedentary: napping, reading, watching TV.

T F 10. The less I move, the less attention I'll call to my body.

95

T F 11. To me, a diet means sacrifice. Something has to hurt.

T F 12. Exercise doesn't work if it doesn't feel like work.

T F 13. I love sports—as long as I'm watching.

T F 14. I wish I liked exercise.

Add up your true answers and false answers:

Exercise Your Passion "true" total: _____

Exercise Your Passion "false" total: _____

If you had more "falses," you're ready to soar. You already have a positive approach to a healthy life and it's only a matter of putting the pieces together to make a consistent, long-term Spark plan.

The more "trues" you had, the more you've been conditioned to treat exercise as a chore—and dieting as deprivation. And yet, there are "sparks" within your negativism. When you aren't thinking about exercise, you'll relish the joy of movement. Listening to music, wanting to dance, feeling the water on your skin—these are all the beginnings of an active life. By starting out slowly and without taking a lot of time or commitment, the Spark plan will help you find your particular motivating Spark and get you not only moving but *wanting* to move.

K's Spark

I've just climbed the stairs of a New York City subway. It wasn't a lot of stairs, maybe twenty in all, but to me that patch of brightness above seemed far away. A man passed me on the left. Another passed, reading a paper. A woman muttered, "Excuse me." They didn't look out of breath; they didn't spend the time from the last stop to this one hoping to make it up the stairs. I'm embarrassed. I'm out of breath. I'm old. And yet I'm only thirty-five. When I was younger, I thought I could burn the candle at both ends, working three jobs, making ends meet, then going out to dinner, socializing. I developed high blood pressure, asthma, gastrointestinal problems. I was a mess.

I didn't know it then, but that trek up the subway stairs, day after day, going from office to office with freelance copy to hand in, would be a symbol of change.

My Spark was smoldering, waiting for something that would catch and flame. There were diets after diets, starvation, liquid, nothing but juice. There were bouts of personal training, gym membership, power walks in the parks. But always they left me cold—and heavier and more out of shape than before.

The Spark wanted to take hold. It wanted to shake me, move me, throw me back into the jitterbug past of shouts and cheers and exhilaration of pure sweat. The stairwell was waiting.

The tests are over and the results are in. It's time to stop contemplating the Spark—and kindle it. In the next few chapters, you'll find out exactly how to kindle your Spark, step by step, day by day, for the next three weeks—and onward.

CHAPTER 4

The Basic Spark Exercise Plan

Lore has it that Abraham Lincoln wrote the first draft of the immortal Gettysburg Address in 10 minutes.

Riding in a machine that goes faster than a horse? Paying bills with a plastic card? Researching the libraries of the world with a click of a mouse? New ideas always seem revolutionary when first voiced. We'll cling to old ways of thinking even if they don't work—until the veneer wears off and that "something new" becomes the norm.

It's the same with the Spark. Although the evidence throughout this book demonstrates that you can do 15 Spark-like bouts of exercise a week and achieve the *same or better* levels of health and fitness as those who go to a gym and work out for a couple of hours once or twice a week, people refuse to believe it. They think you need to feel pain to get fit. They think the more you sweat, the more weight you'll lose. They just can't believe that something so simple, so basic, so mundane as a 10-minute burst of activity can actually make you fit, healthy, and even slimmer.

But it's true. As an exercise physiologist for the past twenty-five

---

SPARK PLUG

Whistle while you work . . . and tap your feet, shake your legs, wave your arms, drum your fingers, and, as demonstrated in a Mayo Clinic study published in the January 1999 issue of *Science*, lose up to 300–350 calories before you turn off your computer for the night.

---

years, I can tell you unequivocally that the Spark program, as unconventional as it may seem, as unorthodox as it may appear, really, truly works.

Don't just take my word for it. Try it out yourself.

K's Spark

It's not like I gave changing my life any thought. It was more like I was still in "wishful-thinking mode." Real change starts out small, with a Spark. In fact, for me, the hard work wasn't the actual change. I didn't even realize it was happening. My hard work came in pushing down the "shoulds."

My first Spark was taking my bicycle out of the garage. Sitting on the seat. Testing the brakes. Trying out the bell. A study in calm concentration, perhaps, to someone walking by but, inside, the shoulds came fast and furious: I should be doing my work. I should return a phone call. I should go to the store.

The second Spark was taking my bicycle down the block. I didn't fall. Even though the shoulds accompanied me past every house, I let them talk amongst themselves.

I ignored their noise and tried a third Spark later the same day—a five-minute ride around my neighborhood. I had begun to change my life and I didn't even know it.

THE 10-MINUTE AEROBIC SPARK
FROM START TO FINISH

To get all the benefits of a 10-minute aerobic spark, you don't need an elaborate, expensive heart rate monitor. In fact, the only piece of exercise equipment you'll use every time you Spark is the *Feeling the Spark: Aerobics* chart below.

It is the primer for my plan, the yardstick for your improved fitness and gradual weight loss. It will ensure that you are not "wasting" your 10 minutes, that you are getting everything out of your Spark. *Feeling the Spark* determines your intensity from the way you feel by using a scale from 1 to 5. As you do your 10-minute Spark, you'll work up from a warm-up level (a 1 or 2) to a strong and steady aerobic tempo (a 3 or 4), then back on down to a 1 or 2 for your cool-down. All within 10 minutes!

Just check to make sure you're within these guidelines and you'll be igniting your Spark within minutes:

Feeling the Spark: Aerobics

Intensity Level	How It Should Feel
1	Gathering Twigs
	Very light, easy. You barely notice anything. Similar to reaching for the remote control to adjust the volume on the TV. Brushing your teeth. Turning the pages of a magazine.
2	Light My Fire
	Warm-up time and cool-down pace. You've gotten off the couch and are approaching the front door. It's the

casual dog-walking pace, the nice-and-easy browsing in a bookstore, the turn at the end of an aisle in the supermarket.

3   Getting Hot
       Brisk, aerobic pace. Slightly faster. More breathing, less conversation. You're walking quickly down the street to make an appointment. Jogging from your car in the parking lot to the office building. Playing doubles in tennis.

4   Soaring Flame
       Hard effort: You're at the peak of your Spark. Conversation in grunts. You don't want to talk! You're rushing to catch the bus. Running for a golf ball in a far-off sand trap. Doing the lindy at a wedding. Exhilaration through the exertion.

5   Inferno
       Too much: You're at 100 percent capacity. Can barely stand, forget about talking. Gasping for air. Running away from a hornet's nest.

During a typical aerobic Spark, as your intensity changes, as you move those arms and legs, you'll ask yourself: "How am I doing? Do I need to push more? Push less?" After the first or second Spark, determining your intensity level with the numbers 1 through 5 will become second nature. After all, measuring how you feel is a lot easier than going to the trouble of taking your pulse—and as accurate to boot.

SPARKLER

"Since I started Sparking, I'm hitting the golf ball twenty to thirty yards farther!"

—NANCY G., a golfer and participant
in the Spark Study 2000

Here's how an aerobic *Feeling the Spark* works, using a 10-minute morning walk in your neighborhood:

1st minute: Stay within 1 and 2 *(Gathering Twigs and Light My Fire)*. You're starting out slow, walking out the door and waving hello to the neighborhood cat.

2nd minute: Stay at 2 *(Light My Fire)*. Go slightly faster. The fence on your right seems to be moving in rhythm with your steps.

3rd minute: Move to 3 *(Getting Hot)*. You've got it. Keep going. A little faster. No time to stop and chat with your neighbor. You couldn't keep up the conversation anyway!

4th–9th minute: Keep between 3 and 4 *(Getting Hot and Soaring Flame)*. Going and gone. You are getting the maximum benefits of the Spark. Faster, faster. Move those legs. Swing those arms. You got it. You're breathing hard. You're working. You can do this. You can handle this. The houses are rushing by. You've walked almost a full circle. You see the neighborhood cat. He's sleeping on his back on the same lawn.

10th minute: Move back down to 2 *(Light My Fire)*. You did it! Slow down now. Begin to walk slower. Take a deep breath. Speak to your Spark buddy. Make sure you can carry on a conversation and your heart has stopped thumping in your chest. Pick up the morning paper and walk back through your front door.

THE BASIC 10-MINUTE STRENGTH-TRAINING SPARK FROM START TO FINISH

If working out with weights conjures up images of hard bodies in Lycra pumping it up on complicated-looking apparatus, not to worry. My Spark theory also applies to resistance weight training for building

---

SPARK PLUG

A February 2000 report in the *American Journal of Epidemiology* suggests that high-intensity workouts (a level 4 on the Spark scale) are better for health and longevity than a nonvigorous activity. It is also a well-documented observation in exercise physiology that you can get in more high-intensity exercise if you break the total effort into intervals (as in the Spark). The conclusion? The Spark is the best way to get in vigorous exercise without getting wiped out. Even better: The short bursts of the Spark guarantee you'll stick with it longer.

---

muscles and strong bones. In fact, depending on the results of your Spark self-test on strength, at least two (but preferably three or four) of your weekly Sparks will be strength-training exercises to ensure strong bones and toned muscles.

The Spark strength-training exercises will give you excellent results—with nothing more than a nearby clock, the *Feeling the Spark: Strength Training* chart below, and some inexpensive handheld weights. (You can find them in any sporting-goods store selling for as low as 50¢ per pound. My local discount chain sells a set of 3-, 5-, and 8-lb. weights for $15.)

Feeling the Spark: Strength Training

Intensity Level	How It Should Feel
1	Gathering Twigs ***Very light, easy.*** You barely notice anything. Similar to separating white clothes from color.

(continued)

Feeling the Spark: Strength Training (*cont.*)

Intensity Level	How It Should Feel
2	Light My Fire
	Slight weight. You can lift forever. These are the waves you make with your hands lying on a float in the water. Pulling out clothes from a department store rack. Reaching down to tie your shoes.
3	Getting Hot
	A little heavier than normal. You can lift a hand weight or raise a leg 20 times without too much effort. You're bringing the laundry up from the basement. Taking out the garbage. Rocking your baby as you walk from room to room.
4	Soaring Flame
	Hard effort: You're at the peak of your Spark. You can lift a handheld weight 10 to 15 times, but it's tough going at the end. You can do it. You could even push yourself to do 1 or 2 more reps. Toting a carton of books. Carrying two pieces of luggage through the airport. Holding a favorite framed picture up while someone else checks its position on your new living room wall. Exhilaration through the exertion.
5	Inferno
	Too much: You're at 100 percent capacity. You can barely stand, forget about repeating a move. Painful exertion. One or 2 repetitions at the most. Moving a piano. Carrying an air conditioner.

The key to a successful strength-training Spark is to be challenged, but not destroyed. Pushed, but not in pain. Everyone starts at a *level 4, Soaring Flame*. There's no need to warm up or cool down; you can get right into the exercise.

Instead of working toward a higher level of intensity, your goal is a heavier weight. As you become more fit, you simply add more weight, moving from, say, a 3-pound to a 5-pound hand weight, a 5-pound hand weight to an 8-pound one. And, for lower-body and ab exercises that don't use weights, you'll just add more repetitions. (In Chapter 8, you'll find some strength-training exercises you can do with ankle weights as your strength and endurance continue to improve.)

But whatever handheld weight you start with, the Spark strength-training exercises are designed to be as effective as a half hour of reps on a gym's expensive circuit machines.

Just think 4. That's the number you're striving for right from the start—no matter the results of your Spark strength self-test. *Everyone will be at his or her own version of a level 4 intensity. One word of caution: try not to do more than two strength-training Sparks a day.* They'll be more effective if they are spread out through the week.

Here's a typical strength-training Spark, using a 10-minute break in the office. Take off your shoes, make some room on the floor and, if you can, close your door. (I'll show you some more easy strength-training exercises in Chapter 8.)

Note: The following exercises, and all the strength-training exer-

---

SPARKLER

"I definitely see the value of having these weights handy for those 'Sparks'! It has been great to use them as stress busters. My days are really long and extremely demanding and busy, so having the weights close by makes it possible for me to do a quick exercise 'pick-me-up' and then I can go back to whatever I was doing."
—BRENDA M., fifty-two, office manager
and participant in the Spark Study 2000

cises I describe in this book, use a universal 10 to 15 repetitions. As you progress, you might find that you can push yourself further. Instead of increasing your repetitions past 15, *increase your weight*—always staying at your version of a *Feeling the Spark* level 4 intensity. In other words, when a 3-pound weight gets too "easy" at 15 reps, move up to a 5-pound weight, and so on.

1st–2nd minute: Upper-arm strength and toning. Feel the 4 in your biceps as you do the curl.

1. Start with your arms at your sides, body straight, stomach in. Hands should be facing in, gripping weights.
2. Slowly raise your arms up in front of you, to your shoulders, for a count of 2. As you raise them up, turn your arms so that your hands are facing in, toward your chest.
3. Slowly move your arms back down to the original position, again for a count of 2. Start with 10 repetitions, building up to 15 over time. Don't strain.

4. Put down your weights. Rest for a count of 15 to 30 seconds.
5. Repeat the entire sequence.
6. Put down your weights and rest again for 15 to 30 seconds.

3rd–4th minute: More upper-arm work. Make carrying bundles kid's play. Feel the definition in your upper arms, front, back, and side; you will after a few weeks of pressing.

1. Stand straight and tall, this time with your arms bent at the elbow, palms facing out. Hold a weight in each hand.
2. Slowly lift your hands straight up over your head for a count of 2. Palms are still facing out.

3. Slowly lower your arms back down to your shoulders for a count of 2, palms facing out. Repeat 10 times. Push, but don't strain. Build up to 15 over several weeks.
4. Put down your weights. Hang your arms down. Count to 15 to 30 seconds.
5. Repeat the entire exercise.
6. Put down your weights and rest for 15 to 30 seconds.

5th–7th minute: Chair work for strong, defined arms and legs. Don't put away those weights quite yet. Sitting in your office chair, hold a weight in each hand. Inhale. You're about to fly. Feel the 4 soar.

1. Sit on the edge of the chair with your back straight. Feet should be flat on the floor. Rest your weights on the tops of your legs, palms facing in.

2. Slowly lift your elbows (which will lift your arms at the same time) to shoulder height for a count of 2, as if you were un-furling wings. Palms should be facing down.

3. Pause for 2 seconds, then slowly lower your elbows back down to your thighs, palms facing in (again, for a count of 2). The motion looks as if you are slowly "flapping your wings." Repeat 10 times, eventually building up to 15.

4. Put down your weights and rest, still seated, for 15 to 30 seconds.

5. Repeat the entire exercise, including your 15-to-30-second "pit stop."

6. Still seated, clasp your arms across your chest. (This can be done holding weights to your chest, if desired.) Sit up straight, back tall, on the edge of your chair. Feet are still flat on the ground. Inhale. You are about to be "one with your chair."

7. Keeping your arms crossed, come up out of the chair slowly, for a count of 2, and stand. The challenge is to keep your back straight. Only your bottom half, specifically your thighs and buttocks, are working—with a Spark of abdominal tightening, too.

8. Slowly, for a count of 2, move back down into the chair the same way you got up, keeping your back straight, arms crossed. Repeat 10 times, going for 15 over time.

9. Rest, still seated, arms at your side, for 15 to 30 seconds.

10. Repeat the entire chair lift exercise, including your 15-to-30-second rest.

8th–9th minute: Flat stomach time. There's no getting around it. Crunches are the best way to grab abdominal strength, improve your posture, prevent lower back pain, and even make your stomach look flatter. But in Spark time, you only need to do 10 to 15 repetitions to make a difference. And you don't even have to get your suit dirty. You can do your crunches in a chair. Now there's no excuse!

1. No more weights! Sit on the edge of your chair, just as you did in the previous exercises. But this time lean your torso into the back of the chair, as if you were slouching. Your legs should be extended, knees slightly bent, your heels on the floor. Cross your legs at the ankle, right foot over left.

2. Hold on to the sides of the chair, if necessary, for support. Or you can clasp your hands behind your head in true hammock (or chief executive) mode!

3. Look straight ahead, neck and shoulders relaxed. Stomach is tight. Using those abs, inhale and slowly lift your legs up as high as you can without straining your arms or your neck. Stomach only! Hold for a count of 3.

4. Exhale and slowly bring your legs back down to the floor. Go for at least 10 repetitions, building up to 15. Remember, you should only feel a level 4 exertion. If you are fast approaching a 5, stop! More will come as you get stronger.

5. Let go. Uncross your legs. Drop your head and your arms. Really get into that slouch. Count to 15 or 30.

6. Move back into position, crossing your legs again at the ankle, but this time left over right. Hands are clasped behind your head or holding on to the chair. Buttocks are on the edge of the seat, torso is back against the chair. Repeat your 10 to 15 crunches. Rest for another count of 15 to 30.

7. *If you are at home, do these crunches on the floor for optimal results.* Use a mat and wear loose clothing. Legs should be bent, feet firmly on the floor. Hands should be clasped across your chest. Use your ab muscles to crunch up; try to pull your shoulder blades off the floor. Do the same repetitions and

rest periods as with the seated ab crunch; work up to 15 at a time and rest for 15 to 30 seconds in between sets.

10th minute: Strong backs build strong abs. Always balance your ab workout with a back extension. It helps counteract the pull of your abs, prevents injury, and promotes the kind of posture that makes you look slim and confident. To the rhythm of level 4 (*Soaring Flame*), do the "Back Track":

1. Stand tall, in a slight lunge, right foot back and straight, solidly on the floor, left foot forward, knee slightly bent. Arms are at your sides. (For an extra challenge, try doing this holding hand weights.)

2. Exhale. Slowly move your arms straight out, then over your head. At the same time, bend your left knee into as deep a lunge as you can without bending your right leg or taking your right foot off the floor. You are the warrior!

3. Inhale as you slowly return your arms back straight out in front of you, then back to your sides. As you move your arms down, return your left knee to the slightly bent mode of the starting position. (Your right leg continues to be straight.) Repeat 10 times, building up to 15.

4. Change position. This time your left leg is behind you, straight and tall, foot flat on the floor. Your right leg is in front, knee slightly bent. Repeat the exercise 10 times, gradually building up to 15.

5. Bring your legs together, out of the lunge, arms at your side. Take a deep breath. Count to 30. You've just done a complete head-to-toe, top-to-bottom strength-training, energy-producing, stress-reducing Spark—without leaving your office!

K's Spark

I don't know how my husband got me from the bed upstairs all the way down the stairs and outside to the garage in the dead of winter. I had been eating and reading, two of my favorite pastimes. He was so insistent and I didn't want to hurt his feelings. He did buy me the green 28-speed Mt. Pocono all-terrain bike for Christmas.

He grabbed his camera, threw a coat over my shoulders, and literally pushed me out the back door. Our dogs started to bark; we decided to make the "journey" a family affair. Bonnie, the older Westie, got a leash; I carried Doe, the puppy, in my arms.

When D.J. opened the garage door, the bicycle was waiting for me to hop on. My new standard white helmet was hanging over the shiny new handlebars. The bike was so green. So new. So filled with possibilities.

Six months later I rode that same bike 275 miles in three days in the 1998 Boston–New York AIDS Ride.

I wouldn't call that one-minute walk to the garage exercise. I'd call it hope.

THE BASIC 10-MINUTE FLEXIBILITY SPARK FROM START TO FINISH

There are those who think of stretches as "dessert," fluff, the easy stuff after all the work. In fact, many people forget to do them altogether. You know the type: the person in the gym class who likes to get an early start in the shower. The exercise enthusiast who never signs up for yoga because it doesn't burn enough calories. Even you, perhaps, when you've somehow managed to fit in what you thought was a necessary—but time-consuming—40-minute walk.

But, in reality, stretches are a vital component of your workout equation—and they are an integral part of your weekly Spark. Stretches improve your range of motion, enabling you to do more of the things you do every day without strain or injury. They'll keep your back strong and pain-free, as well as help your balance and posture.

Without question, stretches are as much a part of the 1998 American College of Sports Medicine fitness guidelines as aerobics and strength training—and, with the Spark, you'll get the results you want in weeks rather than months!

Need more convincing? There's nothing like a 10-minute flexibility

Spark to provide a much-needed break in the day; it's a burst of relaxation with staying power; it reduces stress, increases energy, and helps you think more clearly.

Now for the best part. You don't have to add a thing. All you have to do is follow the basic Spark plan. Depending on the results of your Spark flexibility self-test, at least two of your 15 weekly 10-minute Sparks are specifically geared for flexibility. These short, fast, but effective yoga-like movements have been designed to go anywhere, at home, on the road, at your desk, even in your bed. All you need is to follow *Feeling the Spark: Flexibility* chart below to ensure you are doing these exercises at an intensity level that feels right—not too taut, not too easy—and you'll be on your way toward a more graceful, stronger body.

Feeling the Spark: Flexibility

Intensity Level	How It Should Feel
1	Gathering Twigs ***No effort at all.*** The only stretch you're doing is the one on the couch. Legs are loose. Arms are resting at your side, your hand's on the remote. You're practically asleep. Riding in a car.
2	Light My Fire ***Slight, easy effort.*** You breathe deeply and softly stretch your body. It feels great. You feel limber. This is the feeling you have when getting a deep-tissue massage. Doing a "cat stretch" in bed, stretching out your arms and legs, then letting them drop. Wiggling your toes right after taking off the shoes you've worn all day.
3	Getting Hot ***A moderate push and reach.*** You can feel these stretches. They aren't strenuous, but they are definitely "in

(continued)

Feeling the Spark: Flexibility (*cont.*)

Intensity Level	How It Should Feel
	your face." You're reaching for a can on a high shelf. Squatting to search for a sweater in your bureau's lowest drawer. Pushing dirt onto a dustpan.
4	Soaring Flame ***Hard effort: You're at the Spark stretch summit.*** You can hold a stretch for half a minute, but you're counting the seconds at the end. You feel a mild discomfort; muscles are tight. Squeezing into a car after a successful shopping trip. Searching for your sock under the bed. Trying to close an overpacked suitcase. It's tough, but it will feel so good when you get there. A feeling of well-being envelops your muscles after the exertion.
5	Inferno ***Too much: You're at 100 percent capacity.*** Your limbs are trembling. You feel a sharp pain after only a few seconds. Straining to reach a shoe under the bed. Trying to do a full split in gymnastics. Reaching for a balloon that got away.

When you think about it, a stretch is second nature. Think of the way you yawn, or move your arms and feet after a hard day's work, or rotate your head to ease the tension. We stretch our bodies all the time and for only one reason: It feels good.

A flexibility Spark is also designed to make you feel good. But it adds structure to your stretches so that you get the maximum benefit from the movement. Performing these stretches will ensure that your *other* Sparks are done at your personal best and are injury-free.

Ideally, flexibility Sparks should be done at your level 3 or 4; each pose should be held for 10 to 30 seconds. However, not every body is limber. The reason can be genetic; some people are just going to make better ballerinas than others. But it's also a matter of lifestyle. If you are sedentary, your body will be a little stiffer, a little less able to stretch. Performing the right number of flexibility Sparks for you (and that depends on how you did on the flexibility self-test) will ensure that you are getting the benefits without the pain. Most likely, the range will be 2 to 4.

A few things to keep in mind when doing flexibility Sparks:

- Try to space your flexibility Sparks throughout the week.
- Stretches are "static" exercises. Do not bounce or lunge while performing them. It is a gentle pull.
- You should feel a steady, continuous contraction only while in the pose. You want to stretch your muscles, not injure them! Stop immediately if you feel a sharp pain, then do the stretch at a lower intensity. (For example, if you're holding on to your ankles and feel a stab of pain, move up to your calves. It's an easier stretch.)

Here's an example of a 10-minute flexibility Spark you can do when you first wake up. (Look for more of my easy stretches in Chapter 8.)

1st minute: Easy-time warm-up. Muscles need to be warm and supple for proper stretching. But you can Spark your muscles with very little effort. You can even warm up in bed when you first wake up.

1. Wiggle your toes and your fingers.
2. Pull your stomach in. Hold for a count of 10 to 30 seconds. Let go. Repeat a few times.
3. Stretch out your arms in one direction, your legs in the other. Hold for a count of 10 to 30 seconds. Release. Repeat a few times.
4. Roll your head gently from side to side.
5. Move your body, doing "snow angels" in the sheets.

2nd–3rd minute: Get a leg up with leg lifts. This exercise works your arms, hamstrings, calves, and lower back. The only "pain"? You have to get out from under the blanket.

1. Lie back in bed. Extend your left leg out long on the bed. Lift your right leg straight up and reach your arms around it, lifting up your head. Clasp your hands behind and just below the knee. (You can bend your knee slightly, if necessary.) Hold for a count of 10, 20, or 30 seconds—whichever feels like a challenging stretch (a level 4) but not a stab of pain.
2. Lower your leg, head, and arms. Relax for 15 seconds.
3. Repeat with your left leg.
4. Relax for 15 seconds.
5. Repeat 2 times on each side.

4th–5th minute: Body twists. You'll be stretching out your hips, your thighs, and your waist with this exercise.

1. Lie in bed, facing up. Bend your knees, your feet flat on the bed.
2. Keeping your knees together, gently roll them to the left. Your head and shoulders are still on the bed, facing up. Hold for 10 to 30 seconds.

3. Gently roll back to the center position, knees bent, feet flat. Relax for 15 seconds.
4. Gently roll to the right. Hold for 10 to 30 seconds.
5. Return to center and hold original position for 15 seconds.
6. Repeat 2 times on each side.

6th–7th minute: Sit and stretch. This exercise limbers up your legs, waist, and spine. One drawback: you have to lift your head off the pillow.

1. Lie flat on the bed, legs long and together, arms at your side.
2. Slowly lift up your upper body, moving your arms down the sides of your legs. Head is loose, looking down. Hold for 10 to 30 seconds.
3. Roll back down to your original position. Close your eyes. Relax for 15 seconds.
4. Repeat 4 times.

8th–9th minute: Rock 'n' rolling. You'll literally be rocking and rolling without getting out of bed with this exercise. You'll also be working your hips, hamstrings, and entire spine to boot.

1. Bend your knees and bring them up to your chest. Clasp them with your arms as best you can. Your head will be lifted up from the bed.
2. Literally rock and roll up and down for 10 to 30 seconds. But keep it slow! You don't want to get dizzy.
3. Let go of your legs. Plop your arms and legs down. Drop your head back down to the pillow. Rest for 15 seconds.
4. Repeat the entire exercise 4 times.

10th minute: A seize the day moment. Take a minute for some reflection. Close your eyes. Take a deep breath in and hold it for 10 seconds. Exhale slowly. Repeat. Feel the warmth throughout your body, how relaxed you feel. Continue to breathe deeply. Picture your-self holding on to this good feeling all day long. Open your eyes. Take another deep breath. You're ready to go!

K's Spark

There's this hill near my block. Bradford Avenue. It's long, steep, and winding. In fact, the incline is so steep that you have to look up, not straight ahead, as soon as you make the right turn onto the street.

But once you reach the top of the hill, it's all a delicious, fast, air-hitting downhill from there.

The first time I tried to get my bicycle up Bradford, I had to stop fifteen times. I know because I counted.

Why was I pedaling up this monstrous hill? It wasn't the thrill of downhill. If I had wanted that, I would have taken up skiing. It wasn't the scenery. The street was lined with monotonous stone walls. Was it stupidity? Sure. And a rock hard, refuse to give in, stubbornness that ignored the blaring horns of cars that wanted to pass me, that pushed past the attractive figure I cut in my baggy, worn T-shirts, cellulite-enhancing bicycle shorts, and bubble-head helmet. But I kept climbing. It was harder each time to start up again, but I refused to get off my bike and walk.

One anemically sunny early morning, while leaning over my handlebars, gasping for breath and waiting for my heart to slow, I pondered why I was doing this. I remembered back to April, just a few months before, when D.J. and I were at my cousin Gail's house for Passover. I had talked to my cousin Steve about the bicycle D.J. had bought me at Christmas. I told him that I'd taken it around the block a few times, but since the cold weather hit, I'd been taking indoor cycling classes at my local Y instead.

Steve told me that if I liked to ride a bike, I should check out the Boston–New York AIDS Ride. I'd have to raise $1,500, but he and his sister Gail, one of the top corporate executives in the country, would help me with pledges. That part, he assured me, was nothing. Then he told me the AIDS Ride consisted of a 275-mile bicycle trek in three days. "A piece of cake," he told me.

Okay. Sure. I checked it out. And received an impressive and inspiring booklet in the mail. And for some reason, I said maybe. Maybe I can do this.

What was it about that AIDS Ride brochure? What in the world made me think that in less than six months I'd be able to pull off 275 miles, many of them on hills that made Bradford look like it was below sea level? Looking back, I think it was that it didn't judge. It didn't tell me I *couldn't* do it. Not then, not before I even started to train, not ever. It didn't say no.

But first, Bradford.

> **SPARK PLUG**
>
> If you think lifting weights won't show up on middle-aged bodies, think again. The average number of biceps curls done in 30 seconds increased by 41 percent in the Spark Study 2000. Chair stands increased by 38 percent in 3 weeks. Sit-ups increased by 77 percent. Darci L., a participant in the study, put it best: *"I never imagined that 10-minute sessions could have an effect. It feels so good!"*

YOUR FIRST SPARK

- 7 to 10 aerobic Sparks
- 2 to 4 strength-training Sparks
- 2 to 4 flexibility Sparks

There you have it. The basic Spark equation. Depending on the results of your Spark self-tests, you'll do an equation that will be an individual mix of aerobic, strength-training, and flexibility Sparks—*but your equation will always equal 15 10-minute Sparks per week.* Sometimes you'll do 3 Sparks a day, sometimes 2 or 1, and sometimes no Sparks at all. (But don't let more than two days go by without *any* Spark.)

But there are Sparks and there are Sparks—and many different ways to get your basic 15:

- ***Did the Spark Launchpad Lifestyle Test show that you crave freedom?*** Check out my *Spontaneous Movement* list in Chapter 8 (p. 186) for aerobic suggestions to get your blood moving and keep your Spark sizzling.

- *Or does your Spark launchpad need structure and routine for takeoff?* Go to Appendix A where you'll find day-by-day sample routines that spell out exactly what you should do and when. You'll find one-page exercise and food menus for Week 1, Week 2, and Week 3 of the Spark plan.

- *And, of course, you are always welcome to combine spontaneous movement with a detailed day-by-day routine.* You just need to get in your 15 Sparks a week—and it doesn't matter how you get there. The important key is to stay Sparked and incorporate them into your lifestyle. Some days you might need the structure of details to keep you motivated; other days, you want no lines drawn in the sand.

- *Think of your flexibility stretches as your quiet time.* Although you only may have to fit in three flexibility Sparks in your weekly Spark equation, you can do more whenever you'd like. Gently rolling your head and stretching your arms and legs in your office after a particularly grueling day. Taking a cross-legged yoga stance and relaxing for five minutes. Doing a few gentle lunges when you first wake up. The Spark *is* your *launchpad,* your fired-up "jet propulsion" to a new, active life. Far be it from me to discourage you from doing more. Go for it!

- *Strength-training exercises can also be individualized.* Feel the satisfaction as you move from a 3-pound weight all the way up to an 8- or 10-pound weight (or more!). As you get stronger, you might even want to take your weights on a walk. And feel free to try any strength-training exercises you see in magazines or on television that "spark" your interest. Just remember: Strive for your level 4 and don't do more than two strength-training Sparks a day.

- ***And I'll be there the whole way.*** In Chapters 6, 7, and 8, I will "walk" you through your entire three weeks on the Spark plan—with day-by-day instructions for both your exercise Sparks and your food Sparks.

There you have it. The exercise plan for the Spark. Safe. Fast. At a level that's at the perfect place for you: medically sound with just the right amount of physical push. And you can get there any way you want!

You might not agree with me that exercise is always fun—but you cannot deny it's doable. Excuses are no longer necessary. Self-sabotage is a thing of the past. Who knows? You might even find yourself looking forward to your 15 Sparks as enthusiastically as a home-cooked meal.

And speaking of meals, you'll find the basic Spark Food Plan in the next chapter.

K's Spark

I knew I'd reached a new level in my fitness Sparks when I dreamed I was in a marathon, racing past the others toward the finish line. I was out of breath, sweaty, and hurting. But I was running. Running! The finish line was in sight. Instead of a wide swath of ribbon, there was a smooth, polished dining room table, filled with platters of food. My family was sitting around it, raising elegant glasses in toast. You did it. Now come eat.

Obviously, when it came to food, my Sparks still had a way to go.

But at least I'd burned off the calories first.

CHAPTER 5

The Basic Spark Food Plan

It took less than 10 minutes for Toulouse-Lautrec, sipping a glass of absinthe, to conceive and sketch his famous Parisian posters, including Moulin Rouge, Jane Avril, and Divan Japonais.

There is diet, and there is dieting. In primitive time, diet was whatever you managed to kill or root out that day. But dieting, or the desire to stay trim, has been around from the time human beings no longer needed to forage to survive. In ancient China, the "new" science of acupuncture has one place a needle in the ear to control appetite. In India, concern over obesity was so prevalent that ancient medical texts suggested ways of reducing it (including one particularly gruesome procedure using testicular tissue). The word *fat* was first used in a negative way at the end of the first millennium, around A.D. 1000.

It took two hundred more years before the desire for small waists led to the invention of corsets in King Edward I's English court, but, by then, the die(t) was cast. Fat, sometimes too much and sometimes too little, was firmly rooted in our consciousness like a genetic fat cell. By the end of the 1800s, housewives bought scales to keep track of their weight, calorie counting took the place of counting pennies, insurance companies made overweight customers pay higher premiums, and the first diet book, by an English casketmaker, who, at 202 pounds, couldn't tie his shoes, became an "instant" best-seller with 58,000 copies in print. That was nothing compared to Dr. Lulu Hunt Peters's 1917 book, *Diet and Health, with Key to the Calories,* the first block-buster diet book published in America—which sold about 900,000 copies.

It wasn't too difficult to see a trend starting: Dieting is good. Dieting is healthy. And dieting is certainly profitable. Eighty years later, dieting is still seen as a panacea to cure everything that ails you. Exercise? Sure, it's important, but it's just not as compelling. Compared to the excitement of the latest diet theory (even if unfounded and steeped in deprivation), exercise is a pale second.

The Spark changes all that, putting things back in the right order. Exercise is vital. Exercise is doable. And exercise, with the Spark soaring inside you, can even be exciting.

But humankind cannot live by activity alone. Exercise might be the "food" of the Spark, but food itself comes in a very close second. The foods you eat, the way you eat them, and how much you eat at one sitting can all influence your health and your weight. The Spark plan is also very much about the foods you consume to make a mighty flame—and this chapter will provide the "soup-to-nuts" details you'll need to soar. Add the Spark Exercise Plan and your body will be fit, firm, and optimally burning fat.

K's Spark

I used to call it a "previous life," the years when I'd been unhap-pily married to someone else. Like so many other women, I sublimated my unhappiness in food: fast foods, gourmet foods, snack foods, any food (as long as it wasn't healthy and didn't take a long time to chew).

Surprisingly (at least to me), when things got really bad right before the divorce, I stopped eating. I had become so miserable, so fearful, that I couldn't even give myself the pleasure I used to get from food.

For one brief moment in time, I was a single-digit clothing size. I was also a single woman. From now on, I'd decided, I no longer had to read diet articles in magazines. I could skip the women's fashions on the sales rack. I could buy a bathing suit with the best of them. And I could eat, and, oh, could I ever, whatever and whenever I wanted.

I was happy. I was free. And I celebrated my happiness the same way I had originally drowned out my despair: with food.

Of course, it didn't take long for my weight to come back. And it wasn't many months after I'd moved into my new studio apartment that I started reading about diets again and I started shopping for beach cover-ups.

It makes sense. I had been on both sides of the same curve. I was either fat or thin, with nothing in between. I hadn't changed my relationship with food. I'd only moved to another town.

It would take another twenty years to reach a point where I wanted to eat healthfully more times than not, where my weight didn't fluctuate from "good" to "bad" and I stopped thinking in those terms.

Where my happiness was no longer wrapped up, tied up, secured and taped, with food.

THE EDIBLE FLAME

There's something I'd like you to do right now. Stop reading. Put down the book. And get something to eat. You heard correctly: eat. Because on the Spark plan, I want you to eat *more*. Of course, that can't mean unlimited chocolate bars and nacho chips and cheese; we haven't figured out a diet yet where huge quantities of these foods won't harm you metabolically or biologically. But I do want you to make healthier choices—and that means carbohydrates. More fruit, more vegetables, more grains, and more legumes (which are another kind of vegetable, in the form of dried beans, lentils, and peas).

And while you're eating more of these "right things," perhaps a slice of whole wheat bread, a bagel, a low-fat bran muffin, a banana, an orange, or even those infamous "dieter's delights" carrot and celery sticks, you'll also be eating the mainstay of the Spark Food Plan: fiber.

Remember the campfire I described in Chapter 2? The best wood to keep a flame soaring and the best way to position those logs for maximum burning power? This is the same principle that makes the **Spark Fuel–Spark Burn** equation work. It's all about the way your body consumes foods and the most efficient way it will burn calories. To briefly recap:

Your "campfire" loves carbohydrates. Your muscles gobble them up quickly. When they are consumed, stored-up fat takes their place to keep the fire burning. Fiber optimizes your ability to burn this accumulated body fat. If you eat fiber-rich carbohydrates, you'll be more easily satiated and you'll naturally crave less fats. By eating less fat and more carbs your body will, by necessity, have to turn more and more to fat storage for fuel. This mechanism occurs when your **Spark Fuel (SF)** is high—and it is the ideal place for weight loss and weight control.

By following the Spark Food Plan, you'll be assured of getting the fiber-rich carbs you need to keep your **SF** high. Combine your high **SF** with the low **Spark Burn (SB),** which you'll get with your exercise Sparks, and you'll have your muscles grabbing at stored fat at an efficient clip—long after you've finished one of your Spark exercises or one of your Spark meals.

THE BASIC SPARK FOOD PLAN

The Spark Food Plan is based on much of what you already know about healthy eating—but with some new, exciting ingredients that I've put to the test in the Spark Study 2000. Many of these discoveries, a culmination of years of research, involve the role of exercise Sparks—and the way they "feed" on your diet. The new truths:

SPARK FOOD TRUTH #1: Fiber Rules

You just can't beat fiber for its heart-healthy, weight-reducing, and energy-producing qualities. It's the crucial component for keeping your **SF** high. As you know from reading this book, I consider fiber almost the "food of the gods"; it's that important to our good health. You'll find fiber in every fruit, every vegetable, and every grain. You'll also find fiber in some proteins: beans, legumes, and nuts.

The Spark Food Plan doesn't count calories. It doesn't count grams. But it does count fiber servings. Ideally, you should have eaten at least 10 servings of fiber, or as I call them, fiber Sparks, at the end of the day. That will give you the minimum 25 grams you'll need for optimal weight loss and a heart-healthy life. Every time you eat something that's high in fiber, jot it down in a notebook, on a piece of paper, even a Post-it. (I've included a blank Spark exercise and fiber log in the

---

SPARK PLUG

A number of studies have shown that a daily 5-to-10-gram increase of fiber-rich foods, such as whole grains, legumes, fruits, and vegetables, will decrease your risk of heart disease, type 2 diabetes, and certain cancers from 19 to 37 percent.

One study in particular, the Nurses' Health Study, published in the *Journal of the American Medical Association* in 1999, found that a 5-gram-per-day increase in cereal fiber alone was associated with a 37 percent lower risk of cardiovascular disease among nearly 69,000 women studied over a ten-year period.

Unfortunately, the typical American diet (and many low-carb diet plans), is woefully low in fiber—with only about half the recommended daily intake.

The Spark Food Plan, on the other hand, *will increase your total fiber intake by at least 10 grams every day—by doing nothing but adding some fruit and vegetables and whole grain breads!*

---

back of this book for you to copy and use to keep track of your fiber Sparks and your aerobic, strength-training, and flexibility Sparks, if you so choose.)

A high-fiber breakfast, including cereal and berries, and a handful of carrots in the middle of the morning give you three fiber servings—close to half of your daily goal.

Fiber is easy to add to your diet. It's a matter of a few simple substitutions and additions. "I made sure I ate breakfast," said Joanne H., a participant in the Spark Study 2000. "Typically a high-fiber cereal and some fruit. Psychologically, it feels better to get off to a good start."

To help you find your fiber fire, here are the Sparkling Foods that are rich in fiber as well as other nutrients:

Sparkling Grains: Breads, Cereal, Rice, and Pasta

When I say to eat more carbohydrates, I'm referring mainly to the complex kind. The simple carbs are simple sugars such as table sugar and honey. Complex carbohydrates are long "chains" (polymers) of hundreds of thousands, or even millions, of simple sugars, and they are found in two forms in our foods: starch, the basic material of grains, and fiber. Choose high-fiber carbohydrates and you'll get a double dose of the Spark benefits of health, energy, and vitality—and a high **SF** to boot.

Some ideas to Spark variety:

Animal crackers
Bagels (whole wheat, raisin, and pumpernickel)
Barley
Bran muffins
Brown rice
Buckwheat pancakes
Cheerios® cereal
Chex® cereals
Corn bran cereal
Corn flakes
Corn tortillas
Cornbread
Couscous
Cracklin' Oat Bran® cereal

Ethnic grains, such as quinoa, amaranth, and basmati rice
Fig Newtons®
Granola
Grape-Nuts® cereal
Oat bran cereals
Oatmeal
Popcorn (air-popped)
Potatoes
Pretzels
Pumpernickel bread
Puffed rice and wheat cereals
Raisin bran cereals
Raisin bread

Rice cakes
Ry-Krisp® crackers
Shredded Wheat cereal
Spinach pasta
Total® cereal
Wheat germ
Wheaties® cereal

Whole grain bread
Whole wheat croutons
Whole wheat frozen waffles
Whole wheat melba toast
Whole wheat pastas
Whole wheat pita breads
Yams

Sparkling Fruits

All fruits are rich in fiber. Even better, most contain essentially no fat. Along with your high **SF** count, you'll also get a good Spark of antioxidants and phytochemicals.

Some ideas to Spark variety:

Apples, especially with skin
Applesauce—natural
Apricots
Asian pears
Bananas
Berries, including
  blackberries, raspberries,
  blueberries, and
  strawberries
Cherries
Clementines
Dried fruit, including
  cranberries, apricots, and
  pineapple
Figs
Grapes

Kiwifruit
Mangoes
Melons, including
  honeydew, cantaloupe,
  Persian, Crenshaw, and
  Galla
Oranges
Papayas
Peaches
Pears, especially with
  skin
Pineapple, raw
Plums
Prunes
Raisins
Watermelon

Sparkling Vegetables

Vegetables are not only low in calories, they're also fiber-dense. In other words, a handful of carrots will fill you up faster than a handful of chips. (They also have much less salt content.) Add their powerful nutrients and low fat, and there's no holding back. Feel free to indulge!

Some ideas to Spark variety:

Acorn squash
Arugula
Asparagus
Avocado
Broccoli
Brussels sprouts
Cabbage
Carrots
Cauliflower
Chinese cabbage
Corn
Cucumbers
Eggplant
Endive
Field greens
Kale

Lettuce, including romaine,
   red-tipped, escarole,
   curly-topped, and iceberg
Onions
Peas
Peppers, including green,
   red, yellow, and jalapeño
Pumpkin
Radicchio
Sauerkraut
Spinach, raw or cooked
String beans, raw or cooked
Summer squash, including
   zucchini, butternut,
   crookneck, and Hubbard
Swiss chard
Tomatoes

Sparkling Protein

Protein usually conjures up a piece of chicken, a juicy steak or burger, an egg at breakfast, tuna fish, or a grilled salmon with dill. You don't think of protein as having much fiber. Fat and cholesterol, yes.

133

SPARKLER

"I'm ready to Spark. I have here in front of me raisin bran and my fruits and vegetables to eat for breakfast and throughout the day for snacks. I think that's pretty good!"
—MARY W., forty-two, a participant in the Spark Study 2000

Calories, yes. But fiber? Well, think again. Legumes—those beans in chili and lentil soup—and nuts are proteins that are loaded with fiber. (True, nuts also are high in fat, but it's the good, unsaturated kind. If you're concerned, eat only one or two handfuls a day.)

Some ideas to Spark variety:

Black beans	Pecans, dry roasted
Cashew nuts, dry roasted	Pinto beans
Garbanzo beans	Soy products
Kidney beans	Sunflower seeds
Lentils	Tofu
Lima beans	Vegetarian baked
Navy beans	beans
Peanuts, dry roasted	Walnuts

To keep you sitting at that high **SF** campfire, forget about monotony. You need diversity to keep your fire fresh. Here are some ways to get in your fiber without taking out the "joy of eating":

- Add slices of microwaved-softened pepper, carrots, onions, broccoli, or mushrooms to your marinara sauce. Serve it over whole wheat pasta and you'll have at least five Spark fibers in one meal!

SPARK PLUG

Although the Spark Food Plan emphasizes fiber-rich complex carbohydrates, it doesn't mean I don't recommend protein. In fact, protein is definitely muscle power—especially when combined with (how did you know?) high-fiber carbs. To ensure a **high SF–low SB** while still getting the vital nutrients from protein, rearrange the plate. Instead of giving meat center stage at a meal, give grains the spotlight. And watch the fat. It can slow down your Spark, making it difficult for your body to burn that fat you eat—and storing it instead. Keep your fire burning brightly by emphasizing fish, eggs, white meat chicken, pork, and turkey, and 98-percent-lean cuts of red meat. Dianne V., a thirty-eight-year-old participant in the Spark Study 2000, did not want to take cholesterol medicine even though her total cholesterol was 246 at the start of the program. "But I eat a lot of veggies. I made them the focus of my meals, not the chicken or fish." *By concentrating on fiber-rich carbs without excluding her protein, Dianne not only dropped her cholesterol levels during the three weeks to 215 (with 90 percent of this drop in LDL, or "bad," cholesterol), but she lost 26 pounds!*

- Try strawberries and wheat germ on your morning oatmeal or yogurt. It will keep your energy high for hours.
- Try freezing grapes, peeled bananas, and raisins for a delicious change of pace.
- Grill slices of eggplant, zucchini, and onions, sprinkled with garlic powder, on your barbecue or indoor grilling machine.
- Add slices of microwaved-softened zucchini, carrots, and yellow squash to a can of heating tomato soup.

- Instead of ordering white rice in a Chinese restaurant, opt for brown.
- Make your next sandwich on whole grain bread instead of white. (Note: Speaking of white bread, it has been much maligned. Check your labels. Some white wheat breads have as much—if not more—fiber than so-called whole wheat brands.)
- Always have fresh vegetables ready to eat. Wash and cut or chop your vegetables ahead of time and store them in the refrigerator for instant eating.
- Ready-to-use produce, such as washed and bagged fresh spinach and baby carrots, literally make salads in seconds. They also make it easy to add vegetables to recipes.
- Substitute whole wheat flour for all-purpose flour in your recipes for muffins, breads, and cookies. Add some chopped fruit or nuts to the mix. *(You'll find Spark recipes for muffins and bread in the back of the book.)*
- Make meatless chili for a delicious dinner that's packed with fiber: Mix cans of red kidney beans and pinto beans (drained) with tomato sauce. Add hot sauce, chopped onions and peppers, chunks of tomato with the skins, and salt to taste. Serve over brown rice and you'll get an extra fiber Spark.

K's Spark

Sometimes I think the reason I signed up for the AIDS Ride is that I thought if I was an "athlete" I could eat anything and everything and still be trim. Clif Bars. Bowls and bowls of pasta. Yummy delicious candy. What I didn't realize was that the more exercise I did, the less important food became to me. Sure, I wanted a treat now and then, but I didn't torture myself over it. In fact, during the ride, I would look at food as fuel for the next mile stretch. What foods would give me the most energy?

I suddenly had respect for food—and for myself.

SPARK FOOD TRUTH #2: Snack Well and Often

The entire concept of the Spark is one of accessibility. The participants in the Spark Study 2000 consistently say how doable the program is, how easy it is to fit Sparks into their everyday life. You've already seen the ease of the Spark food philosophy at work with your fiber tally. Ten fiber Sparks a day is all you need to keep your **SF-SB** equation where it should be for optimal metabolic fitness and weight control.

But the 10 fiber Sparks a day serve another purpose. The more fiber you eat, the less hungry you'll feel. When you do feel hungry, you *will* be hungry. And on the Spark plan that's a signal to eat. Not ignore, not suppress with white-knuckled willpower, but to eat the fiber-rich good stuff. (A whole wheat bagel topped with peanut butter anyone?)

The appetite satiation self-test you took in Chapter 3 (pp. 91–92) helped make you more aware of how hungry you are when you eat. Here's a short recap for easy reference:

Spark Your Appetite Scale: Short List				
1	2	3	4	5
Starving	Hungry	Can go either way	Satisfyingly full	Stuffed

Ideally, you should always eat when hunger starts to nag, not whine or shout. That means listening to your body, striving for a 2 or 3 on the Spark appetite scale.

You should eat until you're full—but not to the point where you have to undo your belt. You should feel good, not stuffed. Nor should you feel deprived, somehow believing that if you leave the table still hungry you'll lose more weight. Statistics show that's just staving off the inevitable "binge"—and getting your **SF-SB** out of whack to boot. On the Spark appetite scale, fullness should feel around a 4.

A **high SF–low SB,** created with high-fiber foods and exercise Sparks, will help maintain this 2 to 4 range of appetite.

Nibbling your way throughout the day will further ensure that you are eating when hungry and stopping when full. In other words, eat frequent, fiber-rich snacks. Try to eat smaller, more frequent meals, and spread them out throughout the day. Studies show that this strategy can lower blood cholesterol and insulin—even without reducing your food intake—and reduce the chances of con-

---

SPARKLER

"Before I Sparked, I would always be so hungry at the end of the day that by the time I got home I would just practically 'inhale' my food. And because I was so hungry I would eat whatever was handy, which was not always the healthiest food. But by eating nutritious snacks during the day, I never let my hunger get too great. Now when I get home at the end of the day, I don't 'pig out.' I'm more inclined to prepare a good, healthy dinner—and I have the energy to do it, too!"

—JOANNE H., fifty, a participant in the Spark Study 2000

---

verting the calories you eat into body fat. This is especially true when the "nibbling way of life" is combined with exercise Spark breaks.

SPARK FOOD TRUTH #3: Size Matters

If you follow the Spark Food Plan, listening to your appetite and nibbling at least 10 fiber Sparks throughout the day, you won't be overeating. Simplicity is key to the Spark, in both exercise and food. Although there is no calorie counting in the Spark, humankind does not live on fiber alone. Protein, dairy, and, yes, oils and sweets are an important component of a healthy daily diet. To lose weight even faster, use Spark sight to control your portions. In other words, eyeball your portions to ensure you aren't eating too much (or too little!) of the foods that tempt you. Trust your Spark sight—and these rough estimates:

- 3 ounces of meat, fish, or poultry equal a deck of cards.
- 1 ounce of cheese equals the size of your thumb.
- 1 cup of pasta, cereal, or rice or one piece of fruit equals the size of your fist.
- 1 tablespoon of sauce or peanut butter equals the size of your thumb.
- 1 teaspoon of oil equals the size of the tip of your thumb.
- 2 ounces of pretzels, nuts, or dried fruit equals your cupped hand.

SPARK FOOD TRUTH #4: Skim the Fat

If you consume too much fat, your **SF-SB** equation will become unhinged. Instead of gobbling up the stored fat that's accumulated over the years, your body will be quite happy, thank you, with the fat you've just enjoyed.

Unfortunately, the cliché is still true: Eating too much fat makes you fat. (One gram of fat equals 9 calories as compared to 1 gram of both protein and carbohydrates—which equal only 4 calories per gram.) But we also know fat can make other foods taste great. The best way to handle fat so you won't gain weight? Eat less fat.

You can be assured of keeping your fat intake down by simply reducing the amount of fat you consume. Here are some of the ways people in the Spark Study 2000 have cut fat successfully. *(You'll find a list of higher-fat foods and their lower-fat alternatives on pp. 142–43.)*

- Grill or broil your meats instead of pan frying them. Brush roasting chicken with chicken broth instead of butter. Trim the fat off your meats after they've cooked (that way you'll be able to "lock in" the flavor and avoid too dry results).
- Don't forgo all the fat in recipes—just cut the ingredients by half or by thirds and see how they taste. Instead of 4 tablespoons of butter, for example, see what muffins and breads and sauces taste like with 2 tablespoons.
- Forget the butter or oil when making pasta, rice, or couscous. There's a reason why it's "optional."
- Use nonstick butter-flavored spray for frying eggs.
- Make yogurt cheese by draining an 8-ounce container of plain yogurt through cheesecloth in your refrigerator overnight. The result is a rich, creamy cream cheese—without the calories.
- Try topping your grilled fish with fresh lemon and plain yogurt and dill instead of butter- and cheese-based sauces.
- Drain off the fat from browned ground meat *before* adding it to other ingredients in a recipe.
- Perk up the taste (and fiber content!) of low-fat cottage cheese by adding pineapple or peaches.

Question: What about sugar? Do I have to stay away from it?

Answer: Technically, simple sugar is a simple carbohydrate. In and of itself, sugar is not "evil." But its frequent partner is. Sugar is usually partnered with fat, particularly saturated or trans fat (hydrogenated or partially-hydrogenated) found in the baked goods, chocolate bars, and "sinful" desserts we sometimes crave. However, used sparingly, sugar can help stave off a binge. If you have an occasional dessert, cookie, or snack, you'll be less inclined to eat the whole bag, plate, or pie.

When you must indulge, don't sacrifice the good taste of *real* foods with supposedly low-calorie, low-fat options. They can be packed with sugar and, in actuality, have almost the same calories as their regular counterparts. Some examples:

Fat-Free or Reduced-Fat Product	Calories	Regular Product	Calories
Reduced-fat peanut butter 2 tablespoons	190	Regular fat peanut butter 2 tablespoons	190
Reduced-fat chocolate chip 1 cookie	128	Regular-fat chocolate chip 1 cookie	136
Fat-free fig cookie 1 cookie	70	Fig cookie 1 cookie	50
Nonfat frozen yogurt ½ cup	190	Regular ice cream ½ cup	180
Reduced-fat ice cream ½ cup	190	Regular ice cream ½ cup	180
Reduced-fat granola cereal ¼ cup	110	Granola cereal ¼ cup	130
Baked tortilla chips 1 ounce	110	Regular tortilla chips 1 ounce	130

Easy Ways to Reduce Fat in Your Diet

Higher-Fat Foods	Lower-Fat Alternatives
Dairy Products	
Evaporated whole milk	Evaporated fat-free (skim) or reduced-fat (2%) milk
Whole milk	Low-fat (1%), reduced-fat (2%), or fat-free (skim) milk
Ice cream	Low-fat or fat-free frozen yogurt, sherbet, sorbet, or ice cream
Whipping cream	Imitation whipping cream or low-fat vanilla yogurt
Sour cream	Plain low-fat yogurt
Cream cheese	Neufchâtel or light cream cheese or fat-free cream cheese
Ricotta cheese	Part-skim ricotta cheese, low-fat cottage cheese
Creamed cottage cheese	Low-fat or fat-free cottage cheese
Cereals, Grains, and Pasta	
Ramen noodles	Rice or noodles (spaghetti, macaroni, etc.)
Pasta with white sauce (Alfredo)	Pasta with red sauce (marinara)
Pasta with cheese sauce	Pasta with vegetables (primavera)
Granola	Bran flakes, crispy rice, etc.
Meat, Fish, and Poultry	
Cold cuts or lunchmeats	Low-fat cold cuts (95 to 97 percent fat-free lunchmeats); fresh lean meat or poultry
Hot dogs (regular)	Lower-fat hot dogs

Bacon or sausage	Canadian bacon or lean ham
Regular ground beef	Extra-lean ground beef, such as ground round, or ground turkey
Oil-packed tuna	Water-packed tuna
Chicken or turkey with skin	Chicken or turkey without skin
Beef (chuck, rib, brisket)	Beef (round, loin), trimmed of external fat

Baked Goods

Croissants, brioches, etc.	Hard French rolls or soft brown 'n' serve rolls
Doughnuts, sweet rolls, muffins, scones, or pastries	English muffins, bagels, reduced-fat or fat-free muffins or scones
Party crackers	Low-fat crackers
Cake (pound, chocolate, yellow)	Cake (angel food, gingerbread)
Cookies	Reduced-fat or fat-free cookies if lower in calories

Snacks and Sweets

Nuts	Popcorn (air-popped or light microwave), fruits, vegetables
Ice cream (cones, bars)	Frozen yogurt, frozen fruit, or chocolate pudding bars
Custards and puddings (made with whole milk)	Custards and puddings (made with skim milk)

Fats, Oils, and Salad Dressings

Regular margarine or butter	Light spread margarines, diet margraine, or whipped butter, tub or squeeze bottle (check trans-fat content)
Regular mayonnaise	Light or diet mayonnaise or mustard

- Whenever a recipe calls for whole milk or cream, use evaporated skim milk instead. It tastes just as creamy without the fat.
- Make a delicious, low-fat salad dressing by drizzling olive oil and good quality balsamic vinegar (the best come from Modena in Italy and, although expensive, are widely available in supermarkets) over your greens. Add salt and pepper to taste.
- Cut the oil in sweet salad dressings by using ½ oil and ½ orange juice or plain yogurt.
- Try plain yogurt with dried chives on your baked potato instead of fattening sour cream.
- Go for part-skim ricotta and mozzarella cheeses. You'll never notice the difference in your Italian recipes.

SPARK FOOD TRUTH #5: Get Milk

Dairy products often get short shrift in our daily diet, even though calcium is so important to the health of our bones. Many people just don't want to give any calories "away" to milk—especially when they dislike the taste of nonfat dairy options.

But the Spark Food Plan recognizes how important calcium is to ward off osteoporosis in postmenopausal women. In fact, the recommended daily intake of calcium for everyone is at least 1,000 milligrams per day, with pregnant and postmenopausal women needing *1,500 milligrams.* (Studies have also found that weight-bearing exercises, such as your strength-training Sparks, will help keep bones strong.)

And the foods that pack the most calcium wallop are dairy products. One cup of milk contains about 300 milligrams calcium, 1 cup of yogurt between 300 and 400 milligrams, 1 ounce of cheese between 150 and 250 milligrams. The problem? Most dairy products are naturally high in fat, especially saturated fat.

The good news is that there are many low- and nonfat products now on the market, providing the same amount of calcium but less of the fat. And many foods (including high-fiber items) besides dairy foods contain calcium. Here are some suggestions to get your calcium requirements in every day without influencing your **SF-SB** equation:

- Use skim-plus milk in your cereal; it has a whole milk taste with skim milk calories.
- Sprinkle low-fat crumbled feta or goat cheese on your salads.
- Eat broccoli. It has 89 milligrams of calcium in 1 cup raw. (And you'll be closer to your 10 fiber Sparks for the day.)
- Shellfish, sardines, and salmon are also rich in calcium.
- Soy products, especially soy milk fortified with calcium, will give you the added plus of natural estrogen as well as all-important fiber.
- Supplements work fine, but be sure you don't overload on them at one time. They can cause gastrointestinal discomfort if you take your daily dose all at once. Calcium citrate supplements are easiest on your stomach.
- And, if pills aren't your thing, chew your calcium supplement with one of the calcium "chocolates" available on your pharmacy shelf; they usually contain 500 milligrams calcium per wrapped chew.

SPARK FOOD TRUTH #6: Tap into Water

I'm not going to say you *have* to drink 8 to 10 glasses of water every day. Some people just have a hard time consuming that much water in a twenty-four-hour period. But I would like you to try to drink as much as you can. By keeping hydrated, you'll help avoid fatigue. Your skin will be less dry. And your metabolism will be working at a healthy clip. This is especially important when you are up to 10-minute Sparks 15 times a week. The more active you are, the more water you need. Some ways to drink up:

- Keep a bottle of water on your desk and sip it during the day.
- Get your water in herbal teas and nonfat broth breaks.
- Keep a bottle of water handy in the car. There's room for a coffee carafe, why not water?
- Go for a seltzer with lime instead of your usual cola.
- Experiment with different waters. Some have fewer minerals than others and have a lighter taste; some have infusions of natural fruit flavor.

K's Spark

Exercise definitely changed my relationship with food. I used to plan meals with the same precision as a wartime strategist. I'd envision my plate, the entrée, side dishes, dessert. "What do you want for dinner?" I'd ask D.J. as soon as he woke up.

But riding my bicycle and training for the AIDS Ride changed all that. The focus was no longer meals; it was going a few miles farther. I ate whatever I wanted, but I didn't want as much. I didn't need the cake every night, the "special treat." By stripping food of its importance, I was able to enjoy it more. I ate when I was hungry and rode my bike when I was doubtful, fearful, or anxious. Food was no longer emotional medicine. It became, for the first time in my life, a real joy. An addition, not a substitution.

And I even lost a few pounds in the transition.

SPARKLER

"It's great to find a diet that treats me like an adult. The Spark Food Plan gives me back the responsibility to eat right. This might sound weird, but it 'trusts' me to eat healthfully. I don't feel like going 'off' it because there's no 'on or off' in the first place."

—NORVA G., a fifty-one-year-old maternity nurse

SPARK FOOD TRUTH #7: Ease into the Spark

Most diets start with their most restrictive plans the first few weeks, believing motivation is higher at the onset and you'll lose more weight (which is mostly water). But the Spark is different. We start out exercising slowly to get our bodies used to it without pain, why not the food? By proceeding at a smaller, more attainable pace, you'll avoid the mood swings and the "white-knuckled desperation" that so often accompany diets that abruptly cut off the fat and sugar you've been eating—and which have perpetuated the idea of diets requiring sacrifice, intense willpower, and an "all or nothing" mentality. The goals first set out in the Spark Food Plan are so attainable that you'll get immediate gratification. And, as we all know, nothing breeds success like success. To that end, as with the exercise Sparks, you'll start your food Sparks slowly, gradually easing into the complete food plan within three weeks. *(You'll find each week completely spelled out, day by day, in the next three chapters.)*

There you have it. The basic tenets of the Spark Food Plan. To recap:

- **Fiber rules.** Get 10 servings of fiber a day to maximize health and weight control.

- *Snack well and often.* Nibble whenever you are *really* hungry.
- *Size matters.* Eyeball portions for maximum weight control.
- *Skim the fat.* Reduce—don't eliminate—the fat you eat. Less is more.
- *Get milk.* You need the calcium for strong bones.
- *Tap into water.* Keep yourself hydrated.
- *Ease into the Spark.* Small steps become big ones. The changes you make that feel comfortable are the changes you'll keep for a lifetime.

There's nothing left to do now but to do it. Whenever you're ready, turn the page and begin your first week on the Spark: the Embers program.

On your mark, get set, and Spark!

CHAPTER 6

Week One: Embers

Master chefs at the legendary Le Cordon Bleu cooking school can whip up a chocolate vacherin, a lighter-than-air confection made of chocolate ice cream and meringue, in 10 minutes. (But it takes only 3 minutes to eat it.)

If you're so out of shape that a two-block walk to the drugstore seems like a mountain trek, if you're a firm believer in George Bernard Shaw's philosophy on exercise—"lie down on the couch until the urge goes away"—congratulations!

Yes. Congratulations. You are the one who will most benefit from the Spark in the shortest period of time.

Starting right now. In your first week on the Spark. Your Embers week. Get ready to move those legs, pump that heart, get the lungs going, the pulse pounding, the face glowing, the blood flowing freely and smoothly through your body . . . in two minutes.

YOUR EXERCISE SPARKS FOR WEEK ONE

DAYS 1 & 2: 2-Minute Sparks

Two minutes? That's it. Two minutes, three times a day for the first two days. Get used to doing a boogie when you hear a great dance song on the radio. Get used to using the stairs to go to the meeting on the floor above you. Get used to stretching your arms above your head and taking a deep breath. Get used to the feel of a 3- or 5-pound weight in your hands. Two minutes: before breakfast, around lunchtime, and early evening.

I know it sounds ridiculous, but think of it: 70 to 80 percent of Americans are not active enough to achieve any health benefits, let alone become fit. That means that millions of people have trouble simply walking around the corner. It's not that the majority of them can't do it physically, it's that they *won't*. They're suffering from inertia, the great enemy of exercise—and a happier life. Start with a two-minute walk, and you'll soon push through your "inertia-affliction." Your heart will begin to pump a little stronger, your circulation will move a little faster, your body will get primed, and your energy will slowly start to emerge from its slumber on the couch. It's all about attitude. If you schedule in 2 minutes of activity, you'll be able to schedule in 3 minutes or 4, until 10 minutes flies by. As Joan K., a participant in the Spark Study 2000, said, *"The Spark makes it just so much easier to fit in exercise now."*

DAYS 3 & 4: 4-Minute Sparks

You're almost at the halfway mark. Increase your Sparks by two more minutes. You'll now be doing four minutes. You can start following a modified Spark, using the *Feeling the Spark: Aerobics* chart (which rates your exertion level from 1 to 5) you first saw in Chapter 4 (pp. 100–01). Here's a "short list" for easy reference:

Feeling the Spark: Short List				
1	2	3	4	5
Almost imperceptible	Fairly easy effort	Moderate effort	Reasonably hard effort	Severe effort

Here's the four-minute aerobic Spark you'll be doing right now:

1st minute: Stay within 1 and 2. Easy does it.
2nd minute: Go to 2 and 3. You're beginning to move a bit more.
3rd minute: Go for it! Aim for 3.
4th minute: Cool-down time. Ease back to 1 and 2.

Smile. You've just done an official aerobic Spark.
Do you need some ideas on how to get in your four-minute Spark?

- The average song is anywhere from 2 to 4 minutes. "Mustang Sally" is 4:02 minutes, "Great Balls of Fire" is 2:03 minutes, and "Respect" is 2:24 minutes. Check the back of a favorite CD; the play time for each track is usually listed.
- Do what Spark Study 2000 participant Nancy G. does: Keep a pair of weights by your computer. While you're waiting for information to download, you can do some arm lifts. In four minutes, you can do at least 4 sets of biceps curls with each arm.
- The average city block is 200 yards. Briskly walk two blocks up, cross the street, and walk back. Complete this circle two times and you'll have your four-minute Spark down in, well, no time.

Remember, an Ember will turn into a flame at its own pace. Trying to forge the fire, fussing over it and stoking it too much, may result in putting it out altogether. I might be stretching the analogy a bit here, but the truth is that you need only to follow the Spark as directed for the good results to ignite. Don't say, "Hey, two minutes? I can jump rope for two minutes, or do jumping jacks, or run on a track. That's nothing!" I guarantee if you push yourself further than the *Feeling the Spark: Aerobics* chart suggests, you'll end up quitting before you've begun. Go slow. No fast, furious bursts. Believe me, you'll be pumping it up just fine.

K's Spark

I remember the first day I realized I had changed. Ironically, it was months after the change itself had actually taken effect. It was a hot day in early June, the day of my first official training ride for the Boston–New York AIDS team. I'd already pedaled Bradford about ten times, crawling to the top of the hill as the sun rose in the sky. I'd pushed myself out of bed (with D.J.'s help) and biked all over Montclair and the neighboring towns in the cool dawn air. I'd even hopped on my bike to do some errands, ignoring the call of my car.

Was I ready? Looking at the group of riders who had gathered on the Manhattan side of the George Washington Bridge, I would have to say, "no way." The thirty-five or so riders were so lean, so confident, so young. I made a conscious effort not to think. I'd already come too far; to stop now would be to admit defeat. I would never have the guts to try again. My Spark would die while I became one with the couch.

I refused to get scared when the leader of the ride read a standard disclaimer before we began. Just the usual. Like how you can die on this ride. I shot a look at the others. No one gulped.

We began. Going through the streets of Manhattan, I was okay. I started to smile. There I was riding up Riverside Drive, the Hudson River to my left, passing people and dogs and baby carriages and parked cars, noticing building details I'd never seen, parks that were greener than I ever imagined; there was even a breeze to cool my face.

This good feeling didn't change until we hit the Palisades Interstate Park on the New Jersey side of the George Washington Bridge. I was smiling until the Hill. The hill they call the Alpine that made Bradford look like the down side of a roller-coaster ride. I kept looking up, craning my neck. The top wasn't any closer. My legs ached. The front of my "figure shaping" T-shirt was soaked with sweat. Everyone else had passed me—except the Sweep. He had to be behind me. That was his job, to ride behind the last person on the ride.

But then I heard the Sweep, Al, the young, twenty-two-year-old, skinny-body-like-a-gazelle Al, talking to my left ear. "You can do it. Go, girl."

The guy was like a gnat, buzzing into that left ear: "Concentrate on your breathing out. The breathing in will take care of itself. Keep your legs moving. Steady. And don't look up the hill. Stare at the concrete in front of your bike."

So that's what I did. I had no choice. My mind was on automatic. Pedal. Breathe. Look down. Pedal. Breathe. Look down. I made it up the Alpine at last before I collapsed. I cried. I wheeled my bike into the rest area where the other riders were gathered, resting, and as I pedaled to a stop, I realized that they were all clapping and cheering. For me. They were congratulating *me*.

153

And that's when it happened, while standing in a rest area, while I shook my head and cried, my whole body trembling. While I looked around at these other people, all with lives, all with issues, all with their own demons, who somehow found it in themselves to cheer for me.

I finally got it. I had changed.

DAYS 5 & 6: 5-Minute Sparks

For the next two days, you'll adjust to doing five-minute Sparks at a clip—half of a full-fledged exercise Spark. Just add an extra minute at the *Feeling the Spark* level 3 or 4.

Feeling the Spark: Short List

1	2	3	4	5
Almost imperceptible	Fairly easy effort	Moderate effort	Reasonably hard effort	Severe effort

---

1st minute: Stay within 1 and 2. Easy does it.
2nd minute: Go to 2 or 3. You're beginning to move a bit more.
3rd–4th minute: Go for it! Aim for 3 or 4.
5th minute: Cool-down time. Ease back to 1.

You should do two or three aerobic Sparks each day, adding, perhaps, another song on the CD or 3 or 4 more blocks on your lunchtime break.

Alternate your aerobics with a five-minute strength-training Spark at your desk or while watching TV, using either 3- or 5-pound weights (or higher if appropriate). Remember that strength-training exercises are always done at your *Feeling the Spark* level 4—which is different for every person. (*Use the same strength-training Sparks you were first introduced to in Chapter 4 or, for variety, check out some different ones in Chapter 8.*)

Here's a strength-training Spark example:

1st–2nd minute: Upper-arm strength and toning. Feel the 4 doing 1 set (10 or 15 repetitions) of biceps curls and 1 set (10 or 15 repetitions) of overhead presses. Rest for 15 to 30 seconds.

3rd minute: Chair work for strong, defined arms and legs. Moving up to an intensity of level 4, do 1 set (10 or 15 repetitions) of a seated fly. Rest for a count of 30 seconds. Then do 1 set of a chair stand. Rest for 15 to 30 seconds.

4th minute: Ab moves. Do 1 set (10 or 15 repetitions) of a seated abdominal crunch. (You can also do this on the floor if you prefer.) Rest for 15 to 30 seconds.

5th minute: Back to backs. Balance your ab work with a back extension, doing 1 set (10 or 15 repetitions) on each leg. Rest for the last few seconds.

Try doing a five-minute stretching Spark right before you go to sleep. Use the flexibility exercises I've outlined in Chapter 4 and Chapter 8, staying at a level that's not too easy, not too tight. You want to stretch, not sear!

Here's a fast five-minute flexibility Spark suggestion you can even do in bed:

1st minute: Easy-time warm-up. Get your muscles ready for their stretch with simple toe and finger wiggling. Tighten and release your stomach, legs, arms, and face.

2nd–3rd minute: Leg up. Do a leg lift stretch on both legs. Extend one leg out long on the bed. Raise the other leg straight up and,

> **Question: What if I go over 10 minutes? Or if I end up doing less? Is it a problem?**
>
> **Answer:** Absolutely not. The key is doing it. Whether 10 minutes, 8 minutes, or 12 minutes, the benefits are there: being active, getting your heart pumping, moving your body. To help you keep track of the "basic 10," simply wear a watch or set a timer. Remember, the Spark plan is not a rigid one. The only way you will make the good things in the Spark part of your life is if it is easily incorporated. Accessible. Fast. Never, ever rigid. Go for the Spark—in 10 minutes (more or less)!

lifting your head up slightly, reach your arms around the leg and clasp your hands behind and just below the knee. Hold for 10 to 30 seconds, bring the leg back down and relax for 15 seconds, then repeat on the other leg.

4th minute: Body twists. Limber up your whole body with a body twist, rolling from side to side. Hold each side position for 15 to 30 seconds. Relax for 15 seconds in between each side.

5th minute: Sweet sleep. Take the last minute of your Spark time for deep relaxation. Close your eyes. Hold your breath for 10 seconds, then release. Repeat . . . until you fall asleep.

Day 7: Relax!

It's appropriate for Day 7 to be a day of rest. Take a second to compliment yourself. You did your first week! How do you feel? I suspect you have a little more energy than when you first started.

SPARK PLUG

When I called Spark study participant Nancy G. to check up on her progress, she told me she'd be going away for a few days. I asked her if she'd be able to follow the program while she's gone. Her response? "Glenn, you designed a great program. Of course I will keep it up!" I told her to forget I asked her that and she went on to say: ***"This is the easiest exercise plan I've ever done in my life. I can Spark anywhere."***

YOUR FOOD SPARKS FOR WEEK ONE

No, I haven't forgotten what you should eat while you're walking and moving and learning what it feels like to become active. The key word here is *should*. There aren't any "shoulds," especially this first week. In fact, you aren't going to change your eating habits that much at all.

DAYS 1 & 2: Add one fruit and two glasses of water each day

In this day and age, most of us *know* what's good for us—and what is not. We know that fried chicken has a lot more fat than skinless chicken on the grill. We know that a chocolate bar is going to have more calories than a carrot. In short, we don't need an education. We *know* what to do.

But do we do it? Like getting off the couch, theory is one thing—and action is another. Only 1 in 4 Americans meet the U.S. dietary recommendations of 3 to 5 servings of vegetables a day and less than 1 in

157

3 meets the recommendation of 2 to 4 servings of fruit. As a result of our poor vegetable and fruit consumption, we consume an average of less than 15 grams of fiber per day—well short of the 20 to 35 grams recommended by the National Cancer Institute. This creates an inefficient **SF-SB** equation, leading to possible weight gain, fatigue, and poor health.

No, change is not easy—unless it's so gradual you're barely aware that you've taken to skim milk, that you feel thirsty because you haven't had eight glasses of water, that you actually order the grilled fish with the sauce on the side because you prefer it. Sound like a dream? Not if you follow the Spark Food Plan, starting today. For the next two days, I don't want you do anything more than add one piece of fruit—your choice—and two glasses of water each day. That's it. You're already making a health change and, along with your two-minute exercise Sparks, starting to gradually shift your **SF-SB** equation to the ranks of the efficient.

SPARKLER

"The most amazing thing about this study, though, was the blood work. To have my cholesterol and triglycerides drop by so much, 246 to 202 for cholesterol and 249 to 168 for triglycerides, in just three weeks is just amazing. I am astonished by this. All the people I have told are also astonished. The program couldn't have been better."

—JOAN K., forty-eight, office worker, mother,
and participant of the Spark Study 2000

DAYS 3, 4, & 5: Add three vegetables each day and one more glass of water

Let's up the ante since you're doing so well. For the next three days, I'd like you to add another glass of water, bringing your total up to three, and three vegetables (along with your one fruit). You can eat your greens any way you choose: cooked, raw, in a salad, in a stew, as long as you eat three servings of vegetables a day. You'll be up to four fiber Sparks daily—well on your way to the fiber Spark basic 10.

DAY 6 & 7: Add one more glass of water, one more fruit, and one more vegetable

It's almost the end of your first week and my guess is you probably aren't giving yourself enough credit for what you've done: you've started to change your life. Not only are you more physically active, but you've taken a more active role in the foods you eat. You've chosen to get more fiber, more vitamins and minerals, more life-sustaining water—by *adding* food to your diet, not taking anything away. Perhaps you drank a full glass of water in the morning when you took your vitamins. Maybe you ordered a side salad with your burger at lunch. And, to satisfy your sweet tooth before going to sleep, perhaps you opted for a juicy Temple orange or a bunch of grapes. You're at six fiber Sparks and going strong.

And, with the help of the Spark Exercise Plan, your dress or pants might fit a little better.

SPARK TAKE, EMBERS: WEEK ONE

Number of aerobic Sparks: _____

Number of strength-training Sparks: _____

Number of flexibility Sparks: _____

Number of fiber Sparks: _____

Weight: _____

I feel: _____

CHAPTER 7

Week Two: Kindling

Alfred Hitchcock's classic *Rope*, featuring James Stewart, was a tour de force of filmmaking. There were absolutely no cuts and, as one reel of film was shot, another was put into the camera. The length of each reel? Ten minutes.

Your second week is beginning and you should be starting to feel the Spark. Creating energy and burning fat with movement. Fueling your muscles with their favorite high-fiber fuel. It might be difficult to believe, but you are on your way to becoming an active, healthy person—like Joan K., one of the participants in the Spark Study 2000. "Exercise was always a *huge* deal," she told me. "Get dressed, head to the gym, take an hour-long aerobics class, then home to shower and change. That's a huge time commitment that I simply cannot accommodate any longer. The Spark is portable, manageable, and effective. Now exercise is spontaneous and a part of my daily routine. Now I have no excuse not to exercise!"

YOUR EXERCISE SPARKS FOR WEEK TWO

DAYS 8 & 9: 6-Minute Sparks

The Spark for this second week is not to move off the couch, but *stay off it.* In other words, you are learning the joys of being active, but you still need to make your Sparks a regular routine, a consistent part of your life. Building up to a basic 10-minute Spark helps reinforce that goal—and in only one more week, make it a reality.

You'll start this second week with a six-minute Spark. To recap your Spark intensity, here once again is the *Feeling the Spark:* short list.

Feeling the Spark: Short List				
1	2	3	4	5
Almost imperceptible	Fairly easy effort	Moderate effort	Reasonably hard effort	Severe effort

For aerobic Sparks:

1st minute: Stay within 1 and 2. Easy does it.
2nd minute: Go to 2 or 3. You're beginning to move a bit more.
3rd minute: Go for it! Aim for 3 or 4.
4th–5th minute: Aim higher. 4.
6th minute: Cool-down time. Ease back to 1 or 2.

Do you need some six-minute inspiration?

• *Add a second track to your CD dance music.* Choose your music beforehand and you won't need to stop to rummage through your collection—or have to wait until the commercial on the radio ends. Best idea? Make a Spark tape of your favorite hits.

- *Leave the "Disco Divas" behind for more unusual music to Spark your dancing soul.* Try African, Latino, Brazilian, gospel, or Louisiana Cajun Zydeco for something different.
- *Pick an area near your home or office that you enjoy, either a peaceful park, a beautiful street filled with trees, or a busy sidewalk with lots to observe.* Wearing a watch with a good second hand or a digital readout, do a Spark walk for three minutes, then turn around and come back the same way. You won't believe how fast the time went.
- *For your six-minute Spark strength-training sessions, just add one minute to your sessions.* Maybe do 2 sets (10 to 15 repetitions each) of overhead presses instead of 1, resting for 15 to 30 seconds in between. Or perhaps 2 sets of seated flies. Or leg lifts. Or feel the burn with sit-ups—at least 10. (If you can, try for 2 sets of ab crunches or sit-ups, 10 to 15 repetitions each.) The choice is yours—as long as you stay at level 4.

K's Spark

Motivation is an inconsistent partner. Sometimes it's determination that gets you moving; sometimes fear. Unfortunately, fear can be perverse. Instead of motivating you to change, it can paralyze you.

The one true motivator that has never failed me is anticipation. When I'm excited about the prospect of something, I'll leap up from the bed, grab a dog, and start dancing. In a writing workshop I took a while back, a teacher described the best way to avoid writer's block: never stop working when you've completed a chapter. Always stop when you still want to work. It will make you eager to begin anew the next day. I've found this philosophy can cross over to every aspect of my life. Exercise. Diet. Love. Always leave them wanting more. You wanting more. If I exercise till I drop, I won't want to go near a sneaker for at least a year. But if I've had a great workout, challenging but exhilarating, I'll be ready to tie my laces and get back into the ring as soon as I can.

Make at least one of your six-minute Sparks a strength-training one during these two days, using 3- or 5-pound weights (or 8-pound weights if the lighter ones seem too easy). Remember, strength-training Sparks are always done at your *Feeling the Spark* level 4— which will feel different for each person. *(You'll find the exercises below described in detail in Chapter 4.)*

For strength-training:

1st–2nd minute: Upper-arm strength and toning. Feel your 4 doing 2 sets (10 or 15 repetitions) of biceps curls on each side. Rest for 15 to 30 seconds between sets.

3rd minute: More upper-arm work. Do overhead presses, using your handheld weights. Do 1 set of 10 or 15 repetitions. Rest for 15 to 30 seconds.

4th–5th minute: Chair work for strong, defined arms and legs. Staying at an intensity of level 4 and holding your weights to your chest, do 2 sets (10 or 15 repetitions each) of a chair stand. Stand for a count of 3. Lower for a count of 3. Rest for 15 to 30 seconds between each set.

6th minute: Move your abs. Try to do at least 10 ab crunches or sit-ups without going higher than a level 4 intensity. Aim for 15 if it feels doable. Rest for 15 to 30 seconds.

SPARKLER

"I think what I like the most is the fact that you can focus on your areas of weakness and choose your own exercises or ones that work better for you. I am trying to do more of the weight lifting and stretching since I have never done any of that and don't need as much focus on the walking, which I do anyway. I also love the fact that the Spark can be fit in just about anywhere. Some days I just try to do the stretching in the morning before I get dressed and walk in the evenings because that works better. I can always lift weights in front of a TV show at night. If I had to find 30 to 40 minutes in one big chunk a day to exercise, it would never happen."

—DARCI L., forty-eight, participant in the Spark Study 2000

Here's a six-minute flexibility Spark to try (at a level 3 or 4) before drifting off to sleep. You can also use it as a revitalizing way to start your day.

1st minute: Easy-time warm-up. Get your muscles ready for their stretch with simple toe and finger wiggling. Tighten and release your stomach, legs, arms, and face.

2nd–3rd minute: Leg up. Do a leg lift stretch on both legs. Hold the position for 10 to 30 seconds each and relax for 15 seconds in between each leg.

4th–5th minute: Sit and stretch. Limber up your spine with a sitting stretch, lifting up your head as you sit up. (Your arms will move down the sides of your legs.) Hold the position for 10 to 30 seconds. Roll your head back down to the pillow and count to 15. Repeat 4 times.

6th minute: Sweet sleep. Take the last minute of your Spark time for deep relaxation. Close your eyes. Hold your breath for 10 seconds, then release for a count of 10. Repeat . . . until you fall asleep. (Or leap out of bed, refreshed, awake, and ready to face the morning.)

DAY 10: 8-Minute Sparks

At 8 minutes, you're still raring to go. Only 2 more minutes to your Spark time and you'll be at the basic 10.

For eight-minute aerobic Sparks:

1st minute: Stay within 1 and 2. Easy does it.

2nd minute: Go to 2 or 3. You're beginning to move a bit more.

3rd minute: Go for it! Aim for 3.

4th–7th minute: Aim higher. You're at 4 and you are moving in the Spark, a Kindling that's sizzling hot.

8th minute: Cool-down time. Ease back to 1 or 2. Take several deep breaths.

For your strength training these three days, simply add more repetitions:

1st–2nd minute: Upper-arm strength and toning. Feel the 4 doing 2 sets (10 or 15 repetitions) of biceps curls. (For variety, try something new. Check out other strength-training exercises in Chapter 8.) Rest for 15 to 30 seconds between sets.

3rd–4th minute: More upper-arm work. Do overhead arm presses, using either a 3- or 5-pound weight, or two filled one-gallon water bottles. Do 2 sets of 10 to 15 repetitions each. Rest for 15 to 30 seconds between each set.

5th–6th minute: Chair work for strong, defined arms and legs. Staying at an intensity of level 4, do 2 sets (10 to 15 repetitions) of a seated fly. Rest for a count of 15 to 30 seconds between each set. Then do 2 sets of a chair stand. Rest for 15 to 30 seconds between each set.

7th minute: Stomach monster. Do 2 sets (10 to 15 repetitions, 20 or 30 total) of abdominal crunches or sit-ups. *(You can also do this sitting in a chair if you prefer.)* Rest for 15 to 30 seconds between each set.

8th minute: Get a strong back. Balance your ab work with a back extension, doing 1 set (10 to 15 repetitions) on each leg. Rest for the last few seconds.

Don't neglect your flexibility Sparks. You'll need them to increase your agility and your range of motion. Use the Spark flexibility exercises I've outlined in Chapters 4 and 8, staying at either a level 3 or 4, one that's not too easy nor too tight. If you feel a "dull ache" as you stretch, that's fine; your muscles are getting "exercise." But if you feel a sharp twinge of pain, stop! That's a sign that you are stretching yourself to the point of injury.

Here's an example of an eight-minute Spark stretch:

1st minute: Easy-time warm-up. Get your muscles ready for their stretch with simple toe and finger wiggling. Tighten and release your stomach, legs, arms, and face.

2nd–3rd minute: Leg up. Do a leg lift stretch on both legs. Hold the position for 10, 20, or 30 seconds and relax for 15 seconds in between each leg.

4th–5th minute: Body twists. Limber up your whole body with a body twist, rolling from side to side. Hold each side position for 10, 20, or 30 seconds. Relax for 15 seconds in between each side. Repeat twice on each side.

6th minute: The sitting stretch. Sitting up, your legs extended, lean forward. Continue moving your torso down, trying to touch your

Question: I always reach a plateau in my diets and my exercise programs. And as soon as I stop progressing, I lose everything I gained—and gain back every pound I lost. Why?

Answer: There's a dearly held belief in our society that if you work hard enough, push hard enough, sacrifice through good and bad times, you'll reach your goals successfully. This might hold true for career and financial aspirations, but as the Spark Study 2000 demonstrates, simple, fast, and doable can work equally as well as more complicated, tougher, time-consuming programs.

If you, like so many others, have worked out long and hard, only to continue to feel fatigued, stiff, and weak, it's possible that you aren't exercising at your optimal level. If you, also like so many others, have cut out your carbs, only to continue to hold on to those "same" ten pounds, it's possible that you aren't eating optimally for you. And if you, like so many yo-yo dieters, find that your weight fluctuates along with your exercise routine, it's possible that you are experiencing "yo-yo fitness," a condition in which you never quite achieve your goals no matter how many exercise and diet plans you try (over and over again).

In other words, if you are moderately fit but stagnant, the Spark can help. By regulating and maintaining your **high SF–low SB** equation with fiber-rich carbs and 10-minute exercise bouts, your body will be on a more even keel. You'll feel satiated faster and longer and you'll have more energy. You'll see continual slow but steady progress—which, most important of all, will give you the positive reinforcement you need to keep going.

head to your knees; your arms will move alongside your body. Hold for a count of 25, then release for 5 seconds. Repeat.

7th minute: The rockabye. This stretch will have you rocking like a baby. Clasping your knees, rock forward and back for 15 seconds. Let go for a count of 15. Then repeat.

7th–8th minute: Quality moment. Take the last minute of your Spark time for deep relaxation. Close your eyes. Hold your breath for 10 seconds, then release. Repeat. Open your eyes and feel ready to face the rest of your day.

DAYS 11 & 12: Do three Sparks every day

The Spark routine is, by now, under your belt. You have it down, from warm-ups to soaring at the height to a nice and easy cool-down. You know your leg lifts, ab crunches, overhead arm presses, biceps curls, and stretches as well as you ever will. You can do the Spark. You are living the Spark. For the next two days, make the Spark even stronger—by committing to doing 3 Sparks every day. As you know, it's not a requirement to do 3 Sparks every day; you only need to do 15 a week to reap the benefits. But for just these two days, I want you to feel the power of the Spark. It will keep you strong in the weeks ahead. You can do this. And who knows? You might end up doing more in the future because you want to, because it feels so good to move.

You can do these three Sparks in any combination you wish, as long as you don't do two of the same strength-training Sparks in one day. (You can do two strength-training Sparks each day, as long as one Spark session concentrates on upper body, including arms, shoulders, and chest, the other on the lower body, including abs, legs, and lower back.)

Some Spark "combo" suggestions:

- 1 early morning "pick-up the paper" walk
  1 upper-body strength training using weights
  1 dance to the radio
- 1 morning stretch
  1 midday stairwell walk
  1 lower-body strength training
- 1 early morning bicycle ride
  1 midday walk
  1 session on an at-home treadmill
- 1 strength-training session with a chair and weights
  1 midafternoon deep-breathing stretch at the desk
  1 jog in the park after work
- 1 morning dance to VH1 while you're getting dressed
  1 walk in the neighborhood
  1 stretch in bed

DAY 13: Rest

You've Sparked hard the past two days and it's time to give your body a day off. Take a nap. Walk your dogs at a slow, leisurely pace. Fill up your car's tank and go for a ride. Let the more efficient metabolic rate you created with your Spark do the work for you.

SPARKLER

"I am up to 15 Sparks and have been so religious about them. I'm delighted with my hand weights!"
—JOAN K., forty-eight, a participant in the Spark Study 2000

K's Spark

If I'd given it any thought, I would have realized that bike riding was my sport, that I had a passion for it. D.J. bought me my green Mt. Pocono and bicycle riding once again entered my life. But I wonder now that I'm on an upswing, now that I've changed my life both physically and mentally, if I will slide again, if I will go back to my old ways. It's so tempting—despite how good I feel, how healthy and invigorated.

Do I succumb? Absolutely. But the difference between the old me and the Karla today is that now I don't stay on the couch. I'll eat more for maybe a day or two, even a few weeks, but then the "new me" becomes tempting, the great way I feel when my muscles are stretched and strong, when my stomach is tight, when my skin is glowing, when my energy is so high there's nothing I can't do.

That's when, if the weather's right, I get on my bike.

DAY 14: 10-Minute Sparks

Believe it or not, you've just completed two full weeks on the Spark plan. Congratulations! Today, and every day from now on, you'll be doing the basic 10-minute Spark, 15 times a week, the only exercise regimen you need for the rest of your life. You should be starting to feel more energetic, stronger, and fit. Chances are your body feels a little more toned; your face is glowing. You can breathe the fresh air a little easier.

Your 10-minute Spark looks like the one you just did on Day 10—and all the days before. You just add two minutes to your routine. For

171

a refresher course on the basics, turn to Chapter 4, where you'll find a recap of the "basic 10" and the *Feeling the Spark* intensity charts for aerobics, strength training, and flexibility. And, to "spark" new ideas for the basic 10, you don't have to go any further than the next chapter, *Week Three: The Fire and Beyond—Finessing the Spark*.

YOUR FOOD SPARKS FOR WEEK TWO

It's always best to gradually add fiber to your diet—which is what you're doing on the Spark. To suddenly eat an additional 20 grams of fiber in a day can mean an upset stomach, bloating, and cramps. That's why in the first week you slowly introduced your body to more fiber and more frequent munching. (Remember the **SF-SB** equation!) This week you'll still move slowly as you incorporate the other *Spark Food Truths* into your diet.

Days 8 & 9: Substitute two high-fiber grains for low-fiber ones and drink two more glasses of water

This is still a transition stage, going from eating everything and anything whenever you want to observing, thinking, and making conscious choices. To that end, and in keeping with the Spark philosophy of easing into change, keep consuming your two fruits and four vegetables—and substitute two high-fiber grains for the ones you usually eat. Typically, Americans have no problem getting in their carbs. But it's usually at the low-fiber end (combined with high fat). All you have to do these two days is merely substitute two better carbohydrate choices for what you usually eat. You can find detailed suggestions for substituting fiber-rich grains and breads into your diet in the *Sparkling Grains* list in Chapter 5. To get you "sparked," here are some more:

- Mix whole wheat pasta *with* your seminola on spaghetti night.
- Eat a bran, carrot, apple-nut, or pumpkin muffin instead of your regular corn or blueberry.
- Make a smoothie snack. Add sliced strawberries, bananas, wheat germ, toasted oat cereal, or granola to yogurt or 1% milk. Add ice, a drop of sweetener, and blend. Your kids will love it too.
- Use whole wheat croutons in your salad.
- Use Grape-Nuts® cereal instead of breadcrumbs before you bake your chicken.
- Try an oat bran English muffin for breakfast.

I'd also like to up the water ante with two more glasses. This brings your total up to six. As a rule, Americans don't get enough water, preferring to drink soft drinks, with all their calories and artificial ingredients. If you drink more water, you'll drink fewer soft drinks. Water will also keep you nice and hydrated (which, in addition to helping your body get the nutrients it needs and eliminate waste more efficiently, means less fatigue, and more supple, healthier-looking skin).

DAYS 10 & 11: Skim the Fat

You've increased your fiber and your water. You're beginning a working knowledge of the Spark's way of healthy eating. But there's

---

SPARKLER

"Amazingly, the vegetables are becoming very easy to work into my eating schedule, and I have always liked fruits and I've started eating more of them."
—BRENDA M., fifty-two, participant in Spark Study 2000

---

still one arena that's crucial for well-being: reducing the saturated fat and the trans fat you eat each day.

Two times each day, either at meals or during your snacks, make a conscious decision to reduce the fat in what you eat. This doesn't mean getting rid of all your fat; you can still enjoy (and should!) a dessert, a sandwich, or a salad dressing if you want it. But, by making predominately healthy choices, the one or two "less than healthy" ones will have diminished impact.

You'll find a "vatful" of suggestions for reducing fat in your diet in *Chapter 5: The Basic Spark Food Plan.* Here are a few more to "spark" your own ideas:

- An apple a day: Use unsweetened applesauce instead of butter in your cake recipes—and unsweetened apple juice as a "meat" stock in soups.
- Order your dressing on the side. Use a fork to dab it on your salad. The smaller portion of dressing will not only taste the same, but you won't end up with wilted greens or that soggy pool of dressing at the bottom of the bowl.
- You probably know that ground turkey makes a lower-fat meat loaf than beef. But how about ground chicken? It, too, has less fat, but it has a more "hearty" taste.
- Try eating whole grain rolls. Their nutty taste is so rich you won't miss the butter. (And you'll be getting a fiber Spark to boot!)
- Use plain mashed potatoes instead of cream to thicken soups, gravies, and sauces. Dilute them with either cooking liquid or plain broth.
- You can have your cake and eat it too. Angel food has the lowest fat of any cake around. Add berries and nonfat whipped

topping and you have a delicious dessert. (Here's a hint: microwave some berries for thirty seconds on high to get a warm, seemingly fattening sauce.)

K's Spark

Vegetables had always been an afterthought in my house, and salads were what you had with the good stuff. We stayed with what was safe: iceberg lettuce cut in chunks, tomatoes, and anything frozen that could be boiled in a bag. No surprise that I grew up with an ambivalence about, if not an outright aversion to, greens.

It wasn't until I met D.J. that I learned to appreciate the green (and red and orange and yellow) stuff. I actually crave salads now. Fresh vegetables. Grilled portobellas, garlic, squash. What's really ironic is that the healthy part of eating vegetables is just a side benefit for me. I eat vegetables because I like them.

Did I really just say that?

DAYS 12 & 13: Refresh Your Hunger Scale

These two days are time for reflection. You're not going to add any foods or water. You are, in effect, going to let the healthy changes you've already made sink in. To recap, as of today, your Spark Food Plan should look like this:

- 4 vegetables
- 2 fruits
- 2 high-fiber grains and breads
- 2 lower-fat substitutions
- 6 glasses of water

It's probably hard to believe you've already added eight fiber Sparks to your diet and that you can drink this much water without floating away. But by gradually making your healthy changes, you've given your body a chance to adjust to this new order.

To help reinforce this new order in your body (and your mind), I'd like for you to use these two days to reflect on how truly hungry you are when you eat.

In other words, before you grab the muffin or the bagel, the second helping of pasta, or even the second handful of baby carrots, ask yourself how hungry you are on the *Spark Your Appetite Scale*, with numbers ranging from 1 to 5. You'll find a detailed *Spark Your Appetite Scale* in Chapter 3 (pp. 91–92), but here, for easy reference, is the short list:

Spark Your Appetite Scale: Short List				
1	2	3	4	5
Starving	Hungry	Can go either way	Satisfyingly full	Stuffed

Try to eat when you are feeling a 2 or 3. Try not to let your hunger pangs go to a 1, starving. You'll grab everything in sight. Eat until you are at around a 4. This is the ideal place for your appetite to be for a maximum **high SF–low SB** equation. It means your muscles are efficiently gobbling those high-fiber, low-fat carbs you're feeding them, while burning some of that accumulated fat.

176

K's Spark

The AIDS Ride was fast approaching. I only had two weeks to go. I still couldn't believe I was attempting a 275-mile bike ride, a three-day journey that was filled with the unknown. I went from thinking "I can do this" to wanting to crawl back into bed and never get up again.

But it was too late to back out now. There were people, friends and family who believed in me, who had donated money so that I could ride. There were the people I'd met on the training rides, people living with AIDS, who knew people who had AIDS, who had people they loved die.

Three days to go and counting.

DAY 14: Add two more high-fiber foods and two glasses of water

Today you start the official fiber 10 by adding two more fiber-rich foods to your Spark. You can mix and match:

- 2 more vegetables
- 2 more fruits
- 2 more high-fiber grains and breads
- 1 veggie and 1 fruit
- 1 high-fiber grain or bread and 1 fruit
- 1 high-fiber grain or bread and 1 vegetable

To "wash down" all that healthy fiber you've started to consume, your water count has also hit the official Spark mark: eight glasses a day. This doesn't mean gulping down three 8-ounce glasses right before you go to sleep. Rather, it means ensuring that you stay well hydrated throughout the day. Keep a bottle of water on your desk. Drink herbal teas. Sip a decaffeinated iced tea in the afternoon. (Caffeine detracts from water's hydration benefits.) Even chicken broth can count as one of your waters (but the high sodium content doesn't make it a number one choice for every day).

You've done it. Achieved a Spark way of life in two weeks. Your smile should be a little brighter; your energy high. Your clothes should feel looser and you might have already lost some weight. Carrying packages might be an easier task. Walking up the stairs might not be accompanied with the usual huffing and puffing. Take a moment and see the "Sparks" of your labor:

SPARK TAKE, EMBERS: WEEK TWO

Number of aerobic Sparks: _____

Number of strength-training Sparks: _____

Number of flexibility Sparks: _____

Number of fiber Sparks: _____

Weight: _____

I feel: _____

The challenge for the third week—and after—will be to simply keep it up. And why not? You've come this far easily enough. There's no reason to think it won't continue. You only have to follow your Spark—and watch the improvements in your health and fitness soar even higher.

SPARKLER

"I felt that I was doing something for myself that I really needed. Even before I learned the results and knew they were positive, I knew it because I felt it physically and psychologically. . . . It's easy and it's effective. You can't ask much more of a fitness program."

—JOAN K., forty-eight, participant in the Spark Study 2000

CHAPTER 8

Week Three: The Fire and Beyond— Finessing the Spark

The universe was created from a series of explosions in deep space that lasted less than 10 minutes.

K's Spark

Spiders don't have anything to do with fitness, but they have everything to do with keeping my particular Spark alive.

You see, like many people, I am really scared of spiders. But they were the furthest thing from my mind the night before the AIDS Ride. The possibility of death, injury, the great unknown, these items took center stage.

So there I was, in Cambridge, at our friends Sylvia and Steve's home, thinking scary thoughts as I lay next to D.J. in the sofabed. I couldn't sleep, even though (or maybe because) I had to be at Northeastern University at 5:00 A.M. for opening ceremonies.

It was time to sleep, but I still stared at the dark ceiling. Would I see my dogs Bonnie and Doe again? Would I see D.J.? Was I crazy after all? I was really scared.

That's when D.J. bent over and whispered in my ear. "You know . . . Doe eats spiders," he said.

"What?" I turned to face him.

"Doe eats spiders. I saw her eating them on the back deck. She pounces on them, rolls over them, throws them up in the air, and gulps them down."

I started to laugh; it grew louder. The image of my silly little Westie puppy gleefully obliterating a spider, the embodiment of all my fear, suddenly struck me as ridiculous. She wasn't afraid of them.

"Doe eats spiders," D.J. whispered to me again the next morning at the university. "Just eats them up." We were holding each other in the dark, crowds of people chattering and talking around us. We both started to cry, then began to laugh. "This is silly. I'll be fine." I grabbed my bicycle, put on my helmet, and said good-bye.

"Doe eats spiders," I said as I went up a particularly steep hill. "Doe eats spiders," I said as person after person passed me on the hill I refused to walk. It became my mantra, my strength, the embodiment of my Spark. If Doe could do it, goddamnit, so could I.

When I asked some of the participants of the Spark Study 2000 what they thought of the program, the feedback was exciting:

"Completely doable," said forty-two-year-old Mary W. **"I felt I was doing something for myself that I really needed."**

"This program has been very helpful in forcing me to stay fit and follow a routine that is neither too difficult nor time consuming," said fifty-six-year-old Ancil C.

"After only two weeks, it's easier going up and down the stairs with my heavy backpack filled with books," said thirty-eight-year-old student Dianne V.

"This program really fits my crazy schedule," said fifty-year-old single mom Joanne H.

"I can't believe what I achieved in only three weeks," said forty-eight-year-old wife and mother Joan K.

The results for the Spark study participants in only 3 weeks were astonishing, as you know not only from reading this book, but from experiencing the Spark firsthand these past two weeks. But there is life during—and after—the first three weeks—and that's where this chapter comes in.

Welcome to the third week—and all the weeks to come—of the Spark plan.

THE FIRE AND BEYOND: EXERCISE SPARKS

You've gone through two weeks, gradually easing into the Spark plan from 2-minute Sparks on your first day of your first week, to the basic 10 in your Kindling week, Week 2. And 10 minutes is where you'll want to stay. You feel empowered, strong, able to almost coast through your day. And the Sparks in this chapter, *Week Three: The Fire*, are designed to keep you that way: healthy, fit, and youthful.

The Fire is the maintenance level of the Spark. It is the basic 10-minute Spark, to be done only 15 times a week, whenever and whatever you choose. It is all the days of the third week and onward. It is the only program that gets you up to speed right away. The Spark has *already* quickly and easily become a part of your daily life—in *less* than three weeks!

To make your Sparks sizzle in the weeks, months, and years to come, here are some suggestions that have been proven to work—and make your Spark even more efficient.

MAKE THE MOST OF YOUR FIRE:
A MORNING SPARK THAT CAN LAST ALL DAY

In the same way that cup of coffee gets your mind going, a morning Spark prepares your body for a healthy, energetic day. Remember that growth hormone (GH) I talked about in Chapter 2? If you do an aerobic Spark within a half hour of getting up, you set the stage not only for an immediate GH surge, but *an amplified GH surge throughout the day*.

Your evening Spark continues to benefit from the Sparks you've done during the day; each Spark feeds on the other. If you are planning to have a large meal at dinner, you might want to choose an aerobic Spark to keep your GH secretion high and your **SF-SB** equation at optimal levels.

Of course, a morning Spark is only a suggestion. You should do your Sparks whenever you want. The key is to do them, and whatever it takes to get you moving, that's great. The 15 weekly 10-minute Sparks alone will ensure you are getting the maximum benefits in your health, your looks, and your life.

THE SUPER SPARK:
AN INTERVAL-TRAINING WORKOUT

You might have thought it was impossible to improve the basic Spark, but there is always room to make things better. In this case, it is the *Super Spark,* a high-intensity, intermittent Spark *within your 10-minute aerobic Spark itself*—which can work as effectively as more traditional interval training in creating a longer-lasting metabolic afterburn, growth hormone (GH) surge, and a more potent **SF-SB** equation. Research at the University of Virginia shows that GH surge is directly related to intensity. The more you pump up the intensity, the more GH you'll release.

Here's what an aerobic Super Spark looks like, using the *Feeling the Spark* intensity chart as a guide:

Feeling the Spark: Short List				
1	2	3	4	5
Almost imperceptible	Fairly easy effort	Moderate effort	Reasonably hard effort	Severe effort

1st minute: Stay within 1 and 2. Warm-up time. You're starting out slow.

2nd minute: Move up to 3. You're getting hot and you're in the Spark.

3rd–4th minute: Go through 4 (just shy of 5's maximum drive). You got it. Keep going. A little faster. A little faster still. You can do it!

5th minute: Ease down to 3. You're still at a brisk pace, whether walking, jogging, dancing, or jumping rope. But it's a little easier. Catch your breath.

6th minute: Ease on down even more, to 2. Nothing to it. But watch out. . . .

7th–9th minute: Move back up to 4 (or just shy of 5's maximum drive). You go now! Going and gone. You are getting the maximum benefits of the intermittent Super Spark. You *are* a Super Spark. Move those legs. Swing those arms. Feel your heart pumping. You're breathing hard. You're working. You got it. You got it now.

10th minute: Move back down to 2 or 1. You did it! Slow down now. Begin to ease back down to normal activity. Take a deep breath. Tell yourself you're a Super Spark as loud as you want.

Here's another Super Spark, using 30-second intervals:

1st minute: Stay within 1 and 2. Warm-up time. You're starting out slow.

2nd minute: Move up to 3. You're getting hot and you're in the Spark.

3rd–5th minute: Move up through 4 (just shy of 5's maximum drive) then back to 3 for 30-second intervals. Give it all you got for 30 seconds. Ease back for the next 30. Back up for 30 seconds. Back down. . . . You'll do this interval a total of 6 times, ending up at 3.

6th minute: Ease down from 3 to 2. Easy does it. But here we go. . . .

7th–9th minute: Move up through 4 (just shy of 5's maximum drive) then back to 3 for 30-second intervals. Again! Give it all you've got. Thirty seconds as intense as you can go. Back on down. Then up again. Then down to 3. . . . In total you are doing 4 intervals and you are getting the maximum benefits of the intermittent Super Spark. You *are* a Super Spark. Feel your heart pumping. You're breathing hard. You're working.

10th minute: Move back down to 2 or 1. You did it! Slow down now. Begin to ease back down to normal intensity. Take a deep breath. Go about the rest of your day as the Super Spark.

SPONTANEOUS MOVEMENT:
SUGGESTIONS FOR AEROBIC SPARKS

Need some ideas to get those legs moving, your heart beating, your body sweating? Here are a few unusual aerobic moves and activities that will not only do the fitness job, but will also prevent boredom from setting in:

African dancing
Badminton
Belly dancing
Hopscotch
Hula hooping
Jumping rope
Kickboxing moves
Martial arts moves
Playing tag with your kids
Racing a Spark buddy a couple of blocks
Racquetball
Sliding boards
Steppers
Swing dancing

GETTING STRONG:
MORE STRENGTH-TRAINING SPARK MOVES

Strength training comes in many shapes and forms. In addition to free weights, there are strengthening bands, at-home equipment, ankle weights, and more. But for an efficient 10-minute Spark designed to work all your major body parts, all you need to do are the exercises I outlined for you in Chapter 4.

For variety, I'm also including a few more strength-training Spark exercises here. They are slightly more challenging than the ones I've outlined for your basic Spark. However, by the time you've reached Week 3, you're ready to meet the challenge. Each one takes approximately two minutes to complete.

You can either substitute one or all of them for your basic strength-training Spark or mix and match, doing only your upper body one day, your lower body the next. And don't stop there. Experiment. Try something new you might see in a magazine. Remember, the Spark is specifically designed to "spark" your good health. If you are motivated to try new moves, by all means do so. Check them out. After all, it's only 10 minutes of your time. But do keep the _Feeling the Spark_ chart in mind. Stay at your version of a level 4.

Calf "Lift-Ups"

Your legs deserve some toning, too. A few weeks of calf raises not only shapes and tones, but also adds power to every step you take.

1. Rest your fingers on the back of a chair that you can comfortably hold with your arms right below your waist. Feet should be flat on the floor. Stand tall, stomach in.
2. Slowly, for a count of 2, move your heels off the floor, still lightly holding the back of the chair for support. Stand on the balls of your feet and your toes for 2 seconds.
3. Slowly, for a count of 2, move your heels back down to the floor. Pause for a count of 2.
4. Do 10 to 15 repetitions. Rest for 15 to 30 seconds, then do another set, if desired.

The Triceps Turn

This exercise works your upper arms, particularly the underside. You'll not only get more definition, you'll also be able to better lift and reach for things.

1. Sit in a chair, feet flat on the floor. Grab your weight with your right hand. Slowly bring your weighted arm up and over your head. Keep the arm close to your head; the right elbow should be above and in front of your right ear.
2. Use your left hand to hold your right arm up as you slowly move your right forearm over and down toward your shoulder blade, as far as you can go without discomfort.
3. Slowly move your right forearm up, above your head to a count of 2; your palm should be facing in; elbow should be close to your ear.
4. Slowly, to a count of 2, bring your right forearm back down behind your shoulder, still using your left hand for support. Pause for a count of 2, then repeat.

5. Do this sequence 8 times, then rest for 15 to 30 seconds.

6. Change arms. Your left arm will now hold the weight and your right hand will support it. Repeat the entire sequence, including the 15 to 30 second rest with the left arm.

Hip Raises

The muscles that work the outside of your hips and thighs help keep you balanced and strong. Stronger hip muscles also mean a better tennis or golf game! Use ankle weights for an extra strengthening jolt.

189

1. Hold on to the back of a chair, feet pointed straight ahead.
2. Slowly lift your right leg out to the side for a count of 3, keeping your foot pointed straight ahead.
3. Slowly move your leg back down to a count of 3. Do 10 to 15 repetitions.
4. Repeat with your left leg.
5. Pause for 15 to 30 seconds. Do another set of 10 to 15 repetitions with each leg.

Question: I've done really well with the Spark. But I want to do more. After three weeks, I'm finding that the 5-pound weights I've been using seem too easy. I'm not sure if I'm getting the best results. My other Sparks are also getting easier. Does this mean that 10-minute Sparks are no longer working? What do I do?

Answer: An important Spark truism: A 10-minute Spark done at the correct intensity will always work. *Always.* My Spark Study 2000 at the University of Virginia unequivocally shows that 10-minute Sparks work. If your workout seems to be less challenging, up the ante, not the time. For strength-training Sparks, replace your 5-pound weight with 8 pounds. (But do start out slowly, perhaps doing only 8 repetitions instead of 15, to avoid injury!) As you continue to improve, you simply increase the weight.

For aerobic Sparks, pepper your 10 minutes with the Super Spark to get your heart pumping faster. (And, of course, I certainly won't try to stop you if you want to take an aerobics class, a spinning class, or a daylong hike!)

And, for flexibility Sparks, hold your stretches for a longer period of time. It might mean doing fewer exercises in one 10-minute session, but it will increase your flexibility and stamina.

In other words, there's a lot of room within a 10-minute Spark to make it challenging. As the cliché says, It's not the quantity but the quality that counts.

Buttocks Tightener

This exercise is designed to make your buttocks and thighs firm by working your gluteus maximus. It will also make your legs stronger.

1. Hold on to the back of a chair, your torso leaning slightly, about 45 degrees, toward the chair. Legs should be straight, feet facing forward.
2. Slowly lift your right leg out behind you to a count of 2. Your torso will straighten as you lift your leg.
3. Hold your leg in the air for a count of 2.

4. Slowly bring the leg back down to a count of 2. Do 10 to 15 repetitions.
5. Rest for 15 to 30 seconds.
6. Repeat entire exercise with your left leg.

GRACE PLUS: MORE FLEXIBILITY SPARK MOVEMENTS

You might enjoy the feel of your muscles when you stretch so much that now a morning or evening flexibility Spark is not enough. You might want to "take 10" in the afternoon, during a particularly stressful day. You might find yourself wanting to sign up for longer "stretches," such as yoga or tai chi classes. You also might become creative, moving your body in ways that make you feel good.

Far be it from me to inhibit your stretching call. Rather, I'm including here some other flexibility exercises that you might want to substitute for your usual flexibility Spark, or incorporate into your own unique 10-minute flexibility Spark. Some are more difficult than the ones I've outlined in Chapter 4. But now, in your third week and beyond, you might want to try them. It's entirely up to you. Each one will take about one to two minutes of Spark time. Remember, as with the strength-training Sparks, do these exercises at *your* perception of a level 4, no more, no less, to ensure benefits without pain.

The Pelvic Rock

You'll feel a nice stretch in your lower body, particularly your buttocks, groin area, and lower back, with this exercise. You'll also build in some strength along with your flexibility.

193

1. Lie faceup on the floor, knees bent, feet flat on the floor. Rest your arms straight down the sides of your body, palms facing down.
2. Slowly raise your torso up off the floor, keeping your head, shoulders, and feet on the floor. Hold for a count of 10 to 30 seconds.
3. Slowly lower your body back down to the floor. Pause for a count of 10 to 30 seconds. Then repeat 2 to 3 times.

The Rag Doll

Ah, the relaxing sensation of letting go. This exercise is aptly called the rag doll because you literally let go of your body as you hang down from your waist. It's a good one to perform at the end of your Spark, after you've stretched your muscles.

1. Stand with your feet pointed straight ahead, arms at your side, knees slightly bent. Take a deep breath.
2. As you exhale, slowly bend your body down from the waist, head loose and hanging down. Try to touch the floor with your fingers or as far down to your ankles or calves as you can reach.

3. Hold for a count of 10 to 30 seconds, then slowly roll your body back up, one vertebra at a time. Your head is the last to come up. Inhale. Wait for a count of 10 to 30 seconds, then do the stretch again. Repeat one more time.

The Cat

You'll feel like a stretching cat as you do this exercise—and as graceful and flexible. This movement stretches out your spine and strengthens your arms and shoulders, too.

1. Get down on all fours, like a cat. Tuck your hips in. Your head should be in alignment with your back, your face down. Slowly inhale and lift your head up. At the same time flatten your

back, arching as if someone put a heavy "cat toy" in the middle of your spine. Hold for a count of 10 to 30 seconds.

2. Exhale, pull in your stomach, and round your back as if there were a giant ball under your body. At the same time, move your head down toward the floor. Hold for a count of 10 to 30 seconds.

3. Inhale and come back to the first position. Count to 10 to 30 seconds, then repeat the whole exercise 2 to 3 times.

The Butterfly

This one is a nice release for your legs and thighs.

1. Sit on the floor and, bending your legs, bring the soles of your feet together. Hold your feet and keep your thighs as close to the floor as possible.
2. Slowly "flutter" your legs for a count of 10 to 30 seconds.
3. Stop the movement and, still holding your feet, try to bring your head down to meet them. Go just as far as you can without pain. Hold for a count of 10 to 30 seconds.
4. Come back to the original position and relax for 10 to 30 beats.
5. Repeat the entire exercise again. Then stretch out your legs, shake them out, and rest for 10 to 30 seconds.

K's Spark

It was one of those moments that knocks you out. At the end of the first day I'd gone almost the entire 100 miles, through Boston and the (hilly) back roads of Connecticut. But the sun was coming down and I was told it was getting too dangerous to ride; I had to get off the road. I was given a foil cover because I was shivering. A sports drink was pushed into my hand and I was ordered to drink. The crew at this particular stop was concerned that I was experiencing heat stroke. They were only looking out for me, but I hated them. They had stopped me from going that last five miles. Worse, they made me get on a bus that was waiting to pick up stragglers and drive them into the first night's camp.

I stumbled up on the bus, muttering under my breath, and was surprised at the number of other riders already seated. Some of them had been on the bus since the last pit stop.

I felt depleted, like a flat bicycle tire. I fell into a seat and gazed out the window. The person sitting behind me tapped me on the shoulder.

I turned around and tried to smile. The woman said, "I just have to tell you. You were such an inspiration to me. I saw you riding up the past few hills and you kept going. All these people passing you, but you stayed put. You didn't get off your bike. You inspired me to keep going. Really. You really are amazing."

A part of me didn't believe her, but the rest of me said, "Hot damn."

I got up the next morning, and after taking my bruised and battered body off the earth, out of the tent, and into the Portosan, I crept to my bicycle.

As I moved the bike out of the field toward the road, I saw the woman from the bus the night before. She was with a guy who was helping her on to a special bicycle. She handed him crutches as she got on the seat. I wanted to go over to her and bow. I wanted to tell her, no, *you* are the inspiration. I wanted to raise her hand high and point and shout to everyone how awesome she was.

But I did none of those things. Instead, I quickly went by without her seeing me. I got on my bicycle, pushed down on the pedals, and started up my first hill of the day.

KEEPING YOUR FOOD SPARK SATISFIED: A DIFFERENT PHILOSOPHY

I could spend the next few pages giving you hints and tips on how to "stay on track," how to keep the weight off, and hold temptation at bay. But there are no secrets and you probably know everything I'd say. After all, you've heard it all before: Order broiled in a restaurant, not deep-fried. Request your salad dressing on the side. Choose fish over sirloin steak most of the time. And seconds? Sure, if you are truly hungry.

No, I won't reiterate the obvious. Besides, you'll find a wealth of information about food consumption throughout the pages of this book. Instead, I am going to give you my take on successful dieting, the one secret that I guarantee will keep you on the Spark Food Plan for the rest of your life.

And the secret is . . .

Don't diet.

I don't mean to be flippant. Rather, I'm trying to make the point of the entire Spark philosophy: It's okay to splurge. The people who maintain a healthy attitude about food regulate their consumption based on internal cues, not the external world of peer pressure, restaurant ambiance, stress, and the mighty "shoulds." They listen to their stomach. They don't continue to eat when they are full. And they exercise. The result? Bodies that naturally correct themselves after an indulgence.

It's true weight control.

Listen to *your* stomach. Forget *your* "shoulds" and eat when you are hungry—and eat what you crave.

Of course, it's better to eat healthfully. I'm not advocating a diet high in fats and sugars. But I am saying that once in a while, if you overdo the fat, if you find desserts calling to you from every corner, it's okay. *As long as you are doing your Spark exercises, you'll be fine.* In fact, as the Spark Study 2000 and other studies show, you will be more than fine. You'll most likely have a higher energy level, feel stronger and more toned, be more optimistic and calm—and be physically healthier to boot!

And if you aren't dieting, there's no diet to go off of, no "good" or "bad" days. Just you and your life.

We all have days that are more stressful than others. Some days, you'll feel more in control. It will be easier to stay within the Spark Food Plan guidelines. But other days it will be more difficult, for whatever the reason. On those days, just make sure you get your Spark exercises in. Don't get white-knuckled. If you need to eat to feel better, do it.

Actually, if you give yourself permission to eat that muffin on the way to work, you'll find that you will, most likely, avoid overeating the entire day. You'll be distracted, not attracted.

THE SPARK FOOD MAINTENANCE PLAN

Now that you know my philosophy, here are my specific recommendations for a lifetime of healthy eating and weight control:

Exercise is diet.

Keep Sparking no matter what. Try to get in your 15 Sparks every week at your *Feeling the Spark* intensity level and you'll keep weight off and the health benefits coming:

- 7 to 10 aerobic Sparks
- 2 to 4 strength-training Sparks
- 2 to 4 flexibility Sparks

Follow the Spark Food Truths the best you can.

Guidelines are just that, guides—not rules, not absolutes. To recap, here are the seven basic tenets of the Spark Food Plan:

1. *Fiber rules.* Eat 10 fiber Sparks each day.
2. *Snack well and often.* Eat according to your internal hunger cues, using the *Spark Your Appetite Scale* (pp. 91–92).
3. *Size matters.* Eyeball your servings.
4. *Skim the fat.*
5. *Get milk.* Consume at least 1,000 milligrams of calcium (1,500 milligrams for postmenopausal women) per day from milk or other food sources.
6. *Tap into water.* At least eight glasses a day.
7. *Ease into the Spark.* Slow but steady wins the, well, you know.

> **When nothing short of a tempting snack will do, opt for a less caloric, healthier one first.**

Yes, there really are snacks that can satisfy that need for something sweet, crunchy, or salty—without sacrificing health or adding extra calories. Here are the snacks I recommended to participants in the Spark study:

- **Pretzels.** True, they are salty, but they are also low in fat—and satisfy that crunch when you need it. The best bet? Organic or whole wheat pretzels made with unsaturated, nonhydrogenated oil. Buying in small bags helps keep your snack from getting out of hand.

- **Fig Newtons®.** Call them a "fiber chip cookie." You'll also get calcium, iron, and potassium in every low-fat bite. Even better: you can buy them in two-cookie "snack" sizes.

- **Frozen fruit bars.** These have the same calories—and the same vitamins and minerals—as a piece of fresh fruit, only they can be more satisfying when you need a "treat." They taste like fruit juice filled with chunks of fresh fruit and come in all varieties: orange, banana, pineapple, strawberry, even mango.

- **Peanuts.** A Harvard University study found that eating only 5 ounces of nuts a week decreases the risk of getting a heart attack by one-third. Peanuts are a good choice because their so-called fatty oil is monounsaturated—with all the same good heart things as olive oil. Dry roasted will keep the fat calories down. For a relatively healthy, completely satisfying crunch, try Planter's Original Peanut Bar®.

- **Chocolate.** Yes, chocolate, at least the dark variety. Studies have found that oleic acid, a monounsaturated fat found in dark chocolate, lowers cholesterol. And dark chocolate is rich in antioxidants to boot. To keep your snacking from getting out of hand, buy a small package of miniatures—and share it with a friend. For a dose of important fiber, dip a strawberry into some of the microwave-melted "good stuff."

💧 *Popcorn.* Three cups of air-popped corn is low in calories and high in fiber. How can you beat it for a sustaining snack—at the movies or at home? If you need some of that "melt in your mouth" taste, buy microwaveable light varieties. You'll get the taste, the quantity, and the same healthy amount of fiber.

💧 *Energy bars.* Although you have to read the labels on these to ensure you're not getting too much sugar or fat, they can provide a satisfying pick-me-up in the middle of the day. Luna® bars, from the makers of Clif® bars, are an excellent choice. They are not only low in calories, but they also contain calcium and soy protein.

💧 *Fudgsicle®.* Get some calcium with your urge to splurge from this classic, low-fat "sherbet on a stick."

💧 **Retake the self-tests in Chapter 3 every few weeks or so.**

To ensure your continued success in the Spark plan, I'd also suggest you take a half hour or so to redo the self-tests, especially at the end of your first three weeks. *Most likely, you will be showing much improvement in aerobic capacity, muscular strength, and flexibility—just as the Spark Study 2000 participants did!*

Just in case your Spark had some wobbly moments, your new results will reignite it all over again. Positive reinforcement is the best match in the world.

K's Spark

I finished the AIDS Ride. I rode down Eighth Avenue in New York City, surrounded by cheering, clapping people.

About two months later, Paul Mickiewicz, the fitness director of my local YMCA, asked me if I had ever thought of teaching.

I stared at him. I shook my head. "Me?"

"Why not?" he said. "I've seen you go from being barely able to pedal in my spinning classes to finishing a 275-mile bike ride. I've seen your enthusiasm and your ability to motivate other people in my classes. With some training here at the Y, I think you'd be great."

Karla, the physical fitness instructor? To me, these were people who were, for the most part, blond, washboard-stomach thin, and most definitely young. They wore Lycra bra tops and neon-colored Lycra shorts. They were, in short, everything I was not.

But Paul believed in me. And I guess, on some level, I believed in myself.

I was fit enough to teach a class.

● Feel proud of the real achievements in life.

Finishing a project, helping your child with his homework, lending a helping hand, saving up for a birthday celebration. These are the times in life that deserve applause; these are the things that bolster confidence, build our self-esteem, and bring us joy. Not the hollow ring of *"I passed up a chocolate bar today, isn't that great?"* It's no wonder that these exercises in rigid self-discipline ultimately fail.

That's it. You've just completed three weeks on the Spark plan. Nothing to it, you say? You're absolutely right.

SPARKLER

"Short exercise segments are now the reality of my life. I lost weight. My cholesterol is down. I feel great!"
—MARY W., forty-two, participant in the Spark Study 2000

K's Spark

So that's where I am right now, teaching classes at my local Y, getting certified as an exercise instructor, and generally living my life. I still remember the AIDS Ride, and I still can't believe I did it.

I still work at changing myself every day. Some days are better than others. Some days I exercise, others I don't. Some days I eat too much, and other times I'm golden.

And I'm still terrified. Before I enter the gym, where seventeen students are waiting for me to teach "Back to Abs" and "Spinning," before I have a meeting, before I go into a room where a party is being held, before there's anything new that I have to face, before each time I get on my green Mt. Pocono bike.

But that's what courage is all about: opening the door, turning on the light, dialing the phone. Getting on my bike. Keeping my Spark alive.

I believe you can change your life. You can make a difference in the way you look and feel. I believe in the Spark—and all that it can do. That first Spark can make a flame.

Joan K. did it, with 100 percent improvement in her muscular endurance.

Pat S. did it, with an aerobic capacity improvement that equals the capacity of someone twenty years younger.

Dianne V. did it, with a weight loss of 26 pounds.

Joan K. did it again, with a drop of 46 points in her total cholesterol levels.

Ancil C. did it, with a rise in HDL or "good" cholesterol of 8.6 percent.

Joanne H. did it, with an increase in flexibility that equals the range of someone twenty to thirty years younger.

These and the other thirty-five participants in the Spark Study 2000 did it—and so can you.

I am committed to getting the Spark message to everyone out there who needs a little push, a little hope, a little Spark, not just to get on with their lives, but to live each day reignited with vigor, strength, and joy.

Try the Spark plan for three weeks and see the difference it can make in your health, your looks, and your life.

This is my promise. This is our promise.

To your Spark.

Glenn A. Gaesser, Ph.D.
Karla R. Dougherty

APPENDIX A

A Week of Spark Sample Exercise and Food Menus

4 Days of Week One: Embers
4 Days of Week Two: Kindling
3 Days of Week Three: The Fire and Beyond

EMBERS: DAYS 1 & 2

EXERCISE SPARKS: 2 MINUTES

It is solved by walking.

—ST. AUGUSTINE

The Good Morning Stretch

1. While still lying in bed on your back, stretch your arms in one direction, your legs in the other. Crinkle up your face. Hold for a count of 10. Release for 15 to 30 seconds.
2. Turn over on your stomach. Repeat the exercise. And release.

Lunchtime Walk

Grab your coat and simply walk for 2 minutes, working up to a level 3. It's taking some effort, but you're not yet breaking into a sweat.

Evening Spark

Turn on the TV. When the commercials start, jump up off the couch and dance to the background music, moving up to a level 3. By the time the commercials end, you'll have done a 2-minute Spark!

EMBERS: DAYS 1 & 2

FOOD SPARKS:
ADD 1 FRUIT AND 2 GLASSES OF WATER

Food is the first thing that loved me back.
— FROM THE OPENING OF THE TV SHOW *RHODA*

Breakfast:

The usual

Snack:

1 orange
Sip a bottle of water at your desk or in the car

Lunch:

The usual suspects

1st Snack:

The usual

2nd Snack:

More of the same

Dinner:

Enjoy . . . the usual
1 glass of sparkling water on ice with a lemon twist

After-Dinner Snack:

Your call

EMBERS: DAYS 3 & 4

EXERCISE SPARKS: 4 MINUTES EACH

Never give in, never, never, never give in.
—WINSTON CHURCHILL

The Good Morning Walk

1. Walk 2 blocks, moving up to a level 3 or 4, stretching your arms up once or twice while you walk.
2. March in place at your front door for 30 seconds to cool down.
3. Take a deep breath.

Lunch Break: Strength-Training Spark

1. Put some quiet music on the radio. Holding on to your hand weights:
2. Do 1 set (10 to 15 repetitions) of overhead presses. Rest for a count of 15 to 30 seconds.
3. Bring weights to your side. Do 1 set (10 to 15 repetitions) biceps curls, one arm per set. Rest for a count of 15 to 30 seconds.
4. Bend over from your waist, arms outstretched behind you, weights still in your hands, legs straight. Do 1 set (10 to 15 repetitions) of triceps curls, lowering your forearms down toward the ground, then back out behind you. Keep your elbows by your sides and your torso in the same bent-over position. Rest for a count of 15 to 30 seconds.

An Evening Dance

1. Put on a favorite dance song—Latino, disco, rock—anything with a good, hard, driving beat. Move furniture (and family!) out of the way, set a timer for 4 minutes, and go!
2. Start on the floor, twisting and moving, for 30 seconds. Move up from level 1 to level 2.
3. Stand up and dance. Sing along for 3 minutes. You should be at level 3 or 4.
4. End up back on the floor, doing a few slow twists, for 30 seconds. Breathe deeply.

EMBERS: DAYS 3 & 4

FOOD SPARKS: ADDING 3 VEGETABLES, 1 FRUIT, AND 3 GLASSES OF WATER

> No man is lonely eating spaghetti—it requires so much attention.
>
> —Christopher Morley

Breakfast:

The usual
1 glass of ice water

Snack:

2 handfuls baby carrots
Sip 1 small bottle of water at your desk

Lunch:

Add lettuce and tomato to your sandwich

1st Snack:

1 apple

2nd Snack:

The usual

Dinner:

The usual
Cooked asparagus
Herbal tea

After-Dinner Snack:

Your choice

KINDLING: DAYS 8 & 9

EXERCISE SPARKS: 6 MINUTES EACH

I am life that wants to live in the midst of other life that wants to live.

—ALBERT SCHWEITZER

The Good Morning 6-Minute Stretch

1. Get your muscles ready with some toe and finger wiggling.
2. Do leg lifts for 2 minutes. Aim for 5 repetitions on each side. Hold for a count of 5 or 10.
3. Put your knees to your chest. Slowly roll your bent legs from one side to the other to a count of 5. Repeat 10 times on each side.
4. Sit and stretch. Try to touch your toes. Hold for 10 to 30 seconds. Repeat.
5. Take a deep breath.

Lunch Break: Beautiful Day Walk

1. Get out your sneakers and head for the local park.
2. Warm up, breathing in the spring air, for 1 minute.
3. Walk at a brisk pace (a level 3 or 4) for 3 minutes. Use the last 2 minutes to cool down and dry away your sweat. Breathe deeply, feeling the sunshine on your face. Head back to the office or your home with a jaunty lift to your steps.

An Evening Interval

1. It's "must see" TV night. Put on your sneakers and grab a jump rope.
2. March in place while you watch the screen during the first set of commercials.
3. Jump rope for a count of 25.

4. March in place for 2 minutes.
5. Jump rope for one more count of 25.
6. March in place for 1 more minute. Start to slow down.
7. Grab some air-popped popcorn and watch the rest of the show from the couch!

KINDLING: DAYS 8 & 9

FOOD SPARKS: SUBSTITUTE 2 HIGH-FIBER GRAINS FOR LOW-FIBER; ADD 2 MORE WATERS

Hunger is not debatable.
—HARRY HOPKINS

Breakfast:

Raisin bran cereal with 1% milk
Strawberries
1 glass of ice water

Snack:

2 handfuls baby carrots
Sip 1 small bottle of water at your desk

Lunch:

Turkey sandwich on whole grain bread
Side salad with olive oil and balsamic vinegar

1st Snack:

1 orange
Decaf cappuccino made with skim milk

2nd Snack:

The usual
Cup of chicken broth

Dinner:

The usual
Cooked broccoli
Herbal tea

After-Dinner Snack:

Your choice

KINDLING: DAYS 10 & 11

EXERCISE SPARKS: 8 MINUTES EACH

> **I do not pray for a lighter load, but a stronger back.**
> —PHILLIPS BROOKS

Upper-Body Morning

1. Put some wake-up music on the radio. Holding on to your hand weights:
2. Do 2 sets (10 to 15 repetitions each) of overhead presses. Rest for a count of 15 to 30 seconds.
3. Bring weights to your side. Do 2 sets (10 to 15 repetitions on each arm) biceps curls. Rest for a count of 15 to 30 seconds.
4. Bend over from your waist, arms outstretched behind you, weights still in your hands, legs straight. Do 2 sets (10 to 15 repetitions) of triceps curls, lowering your forearms down toward the ground, then back out behind you. Keep your elbows by your sides and your torso in the same bent-over position. Rest for a count of 15 to 30 seconds.

Lunch Break: To the Stairs!

1. Get out your sneakers and head for the stairwell.
2. Go up and down 4 floors 2 times.
3. Walk slowly back to your office. No one will even have missed you.

Nighttime Stretch

1. Put on some quiet music. Light a soothing candle. Lie on your back.
2. Slowly stretch your legs in one direction, your arms in the other. Repeat 5 times, holding the stretch for 10, 20, or 30 seconds.
3. Clasp your legs and rock like a baby, up and down. Come up for a count of 10. Try to hold the stretch for 30 seconds. Come down for a count of 10. Repeat 3 times.
4. Do a body twist: bend your legs at your knees and slowly roll your body from side to side. Try to take 20 or 30 seconds to move from side to side. Repeat 3 times.
5. Take a deep breath. Stretch your arms and legs once again. Let go. Sweet dreams!

KINDLING: DAYS 10 & 11

FOOD SPARKS: SUBSTITUTE 2 LOW-FAT ITEMS

Food is an important part of a balanced diet.
— FRAN LEBOWITZ

Breakfast:

Whole wheat toast grilled with low-fat cheese
Sliced tomato
1 glass of ice water

Snack:

1 banana
Sip 1 large bottle of water all day at your desk, in the car, or at home

Lunch:

Caesar salad with grilled chicken; dressing served on the side
Fresh berries
Coffee with skim milk

1st Snack:

Jicama slices

2nd Snack:

Rice cakes
Decaf iced tea

Dinner:

Grilled salmon served with low-fat yogurt and dill sauce
Asparagus

After-Dinner Snack:

Hot-air-popped popcorn
Herbal tea

THE FIRE: DAY 19

EXERCISE SPARKS: 10 MINUTES EACH

Eating alone will not keep a man well; he must also take exercise. For food and exercise, while possessing opposite qualities, yet work together to produce health.

— HIPPOCRATES

Super Spark Sunrise

Open the door and start walking! Do a Super Spark interval walk in the neighborhood:

1. Warm up at a level 2 for 1 minute.
2. Go a little faster: level 3 for 2 minutes.
3. Really move: 30 seconds at a level 4 (almost 5!) and 30 seconds at a level 3 for 3 minutes.
4. Ease up for 1 minute: level 2.
5. Really move again: alternate 30 seconds at level 4 (almost 5!), then 30 seconds at level 3 for 2 minutes.
6. Cool down the last 2 minutes, walking from level 3 to level 2. Go back inside and get dressed.

Tabletop Ten

Sitting at your desk, pick up hand weights. No need to turn off the computer.

- ✔ Do overhead presses for 3 minutes (3 sets, 10 to 15 repetitions each, 15 to 30 seconds in between each set).
- ✔ Biceps curls for 2 minutes (2 sets for each arm, 10 to 15 repetitions each, 15 to 30 seconds in between each set).
- ✔ Triceps curls, hand grabbing one weight behind your head, for 2 minutes (3 sets for each arm, 10 to 15 repetitions each, 15 to 30 seconds in between each set).

    ✔ Seated fly curls for 3 minutes (3 sets, 10 to 15 repetitions each, 15 to 30 seconds in between each set).

Reach for the Stars

1. Reach your arms up over your head. "Climb rope" with your fingers. Hold for 10 to 30 seconds.
2. Bring your arms back down to your shoulders. Cradle your outstretched right arm in the crook of your left. Hold for 10 to 30 seconds, then let go.
3. Move the outstretched right arm near or behind your ear. Bend it at the elbow. Use your left hand to hold the right elbow behind your ear. Hold for 10 to 30 seconds.
4. Bring your arms back down. Repeat with the left arm.
5. Repeat entire stretch 3 times.

THE FIRE: DAY 19

FOOD SPARKS:
10 FIBER SPARKS, 8 WATERS, REDUCE FAT

There is no sincerer love than the love of food.
— GEORGE BERNARD SHAW

Breakfast:

2 Apple Walnut Muffins *(see recipe on p. 247)*
1 orange
Coffee with skim milk
1 glass of ice water

Snack:

String beans
Sip 1 large bottle of water all day at your desk, in the car, or at home.

Lunch:

Smoked turkey sandwich on whole grain roll with lettuce and tomato
Sparkling water
1 apple

1st Snack:

Pretzels

2nd Snack:

1 nonfat blueberry yogurt
Decaf iced tea

Dinner:

Rice and Beans *(see recipe on p. 283)*
Mixed green salad with cherry tomatoes and cucumbers
Dressing on the side
Sparkling water

After-Dinner Snack:

Green grapes
Herbal tea

THE FIRE: DAY 20

EXERCISE SPARKS: 10 MINUTES EACH

> **A man who does not take care of his health is like a mechanic too busy to take care of his tools.**
> —SPANISH PROVERB

Early Morning Bike Ride

Take your bicycle out of the garage. Make sure there is air in the tires. Start pedaling! Ride around the neighborhood. Notice the trees, the sun, and the quiet. Aim for 3 rolling hills in 10 minutes.

10-Minute Strength-Training Boot Camp

1. Place a mat on a cleared floor. And get down!
2. Do 10 to 15 push-ups. Rest for 15 to 30 seconds. Repeat 3 times.
3. Turn over onto your back. Time for sit-ups.
4. Do 10 to 15 ab curls or sit-ups. Rest for 15 to 30 seconds. Repeat 3 times.
5. Still on your back, keep your head flat, and lift up your legs.
6. Using your stomach muscles to hold up your legs, slowly bring them down to a count of 15. Repeat 3 times.
7. Rest! Camp is over for the day.

Sweet Dreams Stretch

1. Lie back on the bed. Stretch your arms and legs in opposite directions. Scrunch up your face. Hold for 10 to 30 seconds. Let go. Rest for 15 to 30 seconds. Repeat 5 times.
2. Bend your knees and clasp them to your chest. Gently rock back and forth for 30 seconds.
3. Let go of your legs, but keep them bent and together. Roll them from side to side for 30 seconds.
4. Hold your bent legs to the right. Twist your upper body in the opposite direction, to the left. Hold for 1 minute.
5. Repeat to the opposite side.
6. Rest for 15 to 30 seconds.
7. Repeat step 1.

THE FIRE: DAY 20

**FOOD SPARKS:
10 FIBER SPARKS, 8 WATERS, REDUCE FAT**

I'm on a seafood diet. I see food and I eat it.
—ANONYMOUS

Breakfast:

Bran Chex® cereal with 1% milk
½ grapefruit
1 glass of ice water

Snack:

1 nonfat lemon yogurt
Sip 1 large bottle of water all day at your desk, in the car, or at home.

Lunch:

Shrimp cocktail
Whole grain roll, plain
Green salad sprinkled with olive oil and balsamic vinegar
Decaf iced tea

1st Snack:

2 Fig Newtons®

2nd Snack:

½ papaya with lime

Dinner:

Broiled Sea Scallops with Ginger *(see recipe on p. 330)*
Asparagus
Baked sweet potato with cholesterol-reducing "buttery" spreads
Mesculin salad sprinkled with olive oil and balsamic vinegar
Fresh berries

After-Dinner Snack:

Hot-air-popped popcorn
Herbal tea

THE FIRE: DAY 21

EXERCISE SPARKS: 10 MINUTES EACH

> **Vitality shows not only in the ability to persist but the ability to start over.**
> —F. SCOTT FITZGERALD

Cat Stretch

Have a few sips of coffee, then stretch in the sun. Get down on all fours. Do a "cat stretch":

- ✔ Make your stomach concave. Bring your head down. Count to 10.
- ✔ Move into an arch, bringing your head up. Count to 10.
- ✔ Go back to the concave position. Repeat 2 more times. Rest for 10 to 30 seconds.

Now add your legs:

- ✔ Make your stomach concave. Bring your head down.
- ✔ Try to bring your right knee in to meet your head. Hold for a count of 5.
- ✔ Then arch, extending your right leg out behind you. Hold for a count of 5.
- ✔ Go back to a concave position, right leg in to bent head. Repeat 2 times with each leg. Return to starting position.

Now add your arms:

- ✔ As you make your stomach concave, right knee bent in, bring your left arm straight out in front of you. As you arch, bring your arm back down to the floor.
- ✔ Repeat arm/leg movement 2 times on each side.

Lunchtime Strengthener: All Ankles

Put on your ankle weights and grab the back of a chair.

- ✔ Do side hip extensions for 3 minutes (2 sets for each leg, 10 to 15 repetitions each, 15 to 30 seconds rest in between each set).
- ✔ Do back hip extensions for 3 minutes (2 sets for each leg, 10 to 15 repetitions each, 15 to 30 seconds rest in between each set).
- ✔ Now sit in the chair. Extend one leg. Hold for a count of 10. Slowly lower your leg back down. Repeat with the other leg (3 sets for each leg, 10 to 15 repetitions each, 15 to 30 seconds rest in between each set).

Musical Evening

Move the furniture and send the family for takeout. Put on a rock classic, Latino, or rap CD or cassette—or turn to a rock station on the radio. Dance in the living room. Dance in the kitchen. Dance up the stairs. Dance, dance, dance—for 10 minutes.

THE FIRE: DAY 21

FOOD SPARKS: 10 FIBER SPARKS, 8 WATERS, REDUCE FAT

Sour, sweet, bitter, pungent, all must be tasted.
—CHINESE PROVERB

Breakfast:

2 frozen nonfat waffles
Sliced strawberries
Coffee with skim milk
1 glass of ice water

Snack:

1 teaspoon peanut butter on 1 slice whole grain bread
Herbal tea

Lunch:

Carrot Soup *(see recipe on p. 228)*
Tuna fish, chopped tomatoes, celery, and lettuce in a whole wheat pita.
Use low-fat mayonnaise
Slice of cantaloupe
Sparkling water

1st Snack:

Cherries

2nd Snack:

2 graham crackers
Decaf latte made with skim milk

Dinner:

Spinach pasta with Vegetable Pasta Sauce *(see recipe on p. 274)*
Arugula salad sprinkled with olive oil and balsamic vinegar

After-Dinner Snack:

Pineapple chunks in its own juice
Slice of Banana Bread *(see recipe on p. 248)*
Herbal tea

APPENDIX B

Spark Recipes

Soups. 226

Salads 237

Breads and Muffins 247

Pasta, Grains, and Beans 262

Main Courses. 296

Vegetables 344

Fruit 355

Desserts 362

Appetizers and Snacks 374

Beef-and-Barley Soup

8 ounces lean beef eye round, cut into ½" cubes

¼ cup all-purpose or whole wheat flour

1½ tablespoons canola oil

2 cups finely chopped onions

½ cup chopped celery

½ cup chopped carrots

1 bay leaf

1½ teaspoons chopped fresh thyme or ½ teaspoon dried

3 tablespoons barley

1 tablespoon reduced-sodium soy sauce

4 cups water or fat-free beef broth

Juice from ½ lemon

Dredge the beef in the flour to coat.

In a large saucepan over medium heat, warm the oil. Add the beef and cook until brown on all sides. Stir in the onions and cook for 5 minutes, or until soft. Stir often to prevent sticking.

Add the celery, carrots, bay leaf, thyme, barley, soy sauce, water or broth, and lemon juice. Reduce the heat to low, cover, and simmer for 1½ hours, or until the beef is tender and the barley is cooked. Skim off and discard any visible fat from the surface of the soup. Remove and discard the bay leaf before serving.

Makes 4 servings

Per serving: 272 calories, 8.4 g fat (28% of calories), 20.7 g protein, 28.2 g carbohydrates, 3.7 g dietary fiber, 39 mg cholesterol, 189 mg sodium

VARIATION:

• *Lamb-and-Barley Soup:* Replace the beef with boneless lamb loin trimmed of all visible fat and cut into ½" cubes.

Cabbage Soup

2 quarts vegetable stock or broth

½ head green cabbage, chopped

1 large onion, chopped

2 bay leaves

Salt and freshly ground black pepper

4 carrots, sliced

6 red potatoes, peeled and cubed

In a large stockpot over medium heat, combine the stock or broth, cabbage, onion, and bay leaves. Bring to a simmer, add salt to taste, and cook for about 30 minutes.

Add the carrots and potatoes and cook for about 30 minutes more, or until the vegetables are tender. Add salt and pepper to taste. Remove and discard the bay leaves.

Makes 9 servings

Per serving: 77 calories, 1 g fat (12% of calories), 13 g carbohydrates, 4 g protein, 3 g dietary fiber, 2 mg cholesterol

Carrot Soup

2 pounds carrots, sliced

1 quart vegetable stock or broth

Salt

½ cup cream or whole milk

1 tablespoon maple syrup

½ teaspoon ground cinnamon

¼ teaspoon ground nutmeg

In a large stockpot over medium-high heat, combine the carrots and stock or broth. Add salt to taste.

Bring to a boil and cook for 20 to 25 minutes, until the carrots are very tender. Remove the pot from the stove and let cool.

In a blender or food processor, puree the carrots in batches with their cooking liquid. Add the cream or milk, syrup, cinnamon, and nutmeg to the last batch. Gently reheat the soup and adjust the seasoning before serving.

Makes 9 servings

Per serving: 101 calories, 1 g fat (1% of calories), 6 g protein, 17 g carbohydrates, 2 g dietary fiber, 0 mg cholesterol

Classic Chicken Noodle Soup

1 large onion, finely chopped

3 cloves garlic, minced

5¼ cups fat-free chicken broth

½ cup sliced celery

⅓ cup sliced carrots

½ teaspoon dried thyme

½ teaspoon dried dill

⅛ teaspoon ground black pepper

4 boneless, skinless chicken breast halves (1 pound), cut into ½" pieces

3 ounces ribbon egg (no-yolk) noodles

1 tablespoon chopped fresh parsley

Coat a large saucepan with cooking spray. Warm the saucepan over medium heat. Add the onions and garlic and sauté for 3 minutes, or until the onions are soft. Add the broth, celery, carrots, thyme, dill, and pepper. Bring to a boil over medium heat.

Add the chicken and noodles and cook for 8 to 10 minutes, or until both are tender. Stir in the parsley. Serve hot.

Makes 4 servings

Per serving: 218 calories, 2.9 g fat (12% of calories), 28.1 g protein, 19.3 g carbohydrates, 1.8 g dietary fiber, 52 mg cholesterol, 508 mg sodium

NOTE:
- If you prefer the noodles done separately, cook them for 8 to 10 minutes in a large pot of boiling water. Drain. To serve, place the noodles in individual soup bowls and top with the hot soup.

VARIATION
- *Chunky Chicken-Vegetable Soup:* Replace 1 cup of the broth with 1 cup canned tomatoes. Chop the tomatoes and add to the soup along with ¼ cup finely chopped green or red bell peppers, ½ cup fresh or frozen corn, and ½ cup quartered and sliced zucchini.

Chicken Gumbo

3 cups water

2 cups fat-free chicken broth

1 small smoked ham bone or 2 medium smoked pork hocks, trimmed of all visible fat (about 1 pound total)

2 small boneless, skinless chicken breast halves (about 5½ ounces total)

2 cups frozen black-eyed peas

½ cup coarsely chopped red or green bell peppers

¼ cup chopped fresh parsley

¼ cup rice

3 large scallions, sliced

1 onion, chopped

1 rib celery, sliced

2 cloves garlic, minced

¼ teaspoon dried thyme

1½ cups reduced-sodium stewed tomatoes (with juice)

¾ cup sliced fresh or frozen okra

⅛ teaspoon ground black pepper

⅛ teaspoon ground red pepper (optional)

In a Dutch oven or large saucepan, combine the water, broth, ham bone or pork hocks, chicken, black-eyed peas, bell peppers, parsley, rice, scallions, onions, celery, garlic, and thyme. Bring to a boil over medium-high heat. Reduce the heat, cover, and simmer, stirring occasionally, for 20 minutes.

Using tongs, remove the chicken and transfer it to a plate to cool. Simmer the gumbo for 10 minutes more.

Stir in the tomatoes (with juice), okra, black pepper, and red pepper (if using). Cover and simmer, stirring occasionally, for 10 minutes.

Meanwhile, cut the chicken into bite-size pieces. Add the chicken to the pan. Remove and discard the ham bone or pork hocks. Skim off and discard any visible fat from the surface of the mixture. Simmer for 5 minutes, or just until the chicken is heated through.

Makes 4 servings

Per serving: 295 calories, 4 g fat (12% of calories), 23.2 g protein, 43.3 g carbohydrates, 7.5 g dietary fiber, 34 mg cholesterol, 324 mg sodium

Corn Chowder

1½ cups fat-free chicken broth

1½ cups water

1 baking potato, peeled and finely chopped

1 onion, finely chopped

1 small clove garlic, minced

½ teaspoon dried thyme

¼ teaspoon ground black pepper

⅛ teaspoon dried basil

1½ cups fresh or frozen corn

½ cup finely chopped red bell pepper

1 small zucchini, finely chopped

½ cup fat-free evaporated milk

In a large saucepan over medium-high heat, bring the broth, water, potatoes, onions, garlic, thyme, pepper, and basil to a boil. Cook for 10 minutes, or until the potatoes are tender.

Let cool for a few minutes, than ladle half of the vegetables and about 1 cup of the liquid into a food processor or blender. Add ½ cup of the corn. Process until coarsely pureed. Return to the saucepan.

Stir in the red peppers, zucchini, and remaining 1 cup corn. Cook over medium heat for 8 minutes, or until the zucchini is tender. Stir in the milk and warm through.

Makes 4 servings

Per serving: 144 calories, 0.4 g fat (2% of calories), 7.9 g protein, 30.5 g carbohydrates, 3.3 g dietary fiber, 1 mg cholesterol, 170 mg sodium

Cream of Broccoli Soup

1 small head broccoli (about 1 pound)

1 tablespoon canola oil

1 cup sliced leeks (white part only)

½ cup sliced celery

4 cups fat-free chicken broth

2 cups fat-free evaporated milk

¼ cup cornstarch

1 teaspoon chopped fresh thyme

⅛ teaspoon ground black pepper

Cut the broccoli into florets and set aside. Trim and discard the tough fibrous skin from the stems. Coarsely chop the stems and set aside.

In a medium saucepan over medium-low heat, warm the oil. Add the leeks and celery and sauté for 8 minutes, or until the leeks are soft. Add the broccoli stems and broth. Bring to a boil, then reduce the heat to low, cover and simmer for 15 minutes. Add the broccoli florets and simmer for 10 minutes more.

Puree the mixture in a food processor or blender. Return to the saucepan.

Meanwhile, in a small bowl, whisk together ¼ cup of the milk and the cornstarch until smooth. Slowly add to the broccoli mixture, stirring constantly, over medium heat. Stir in the remaining 1¾ cups milk, thyme, and pepper. Cook and stir until thickened and bubbly. Cook and stir for 2 minutes more.

Makes 4 servings

Per serving: 233 calories, 4.1 g fat (15% of calories), 17.8 g protein, 32.9 g carbohydrates, 0.9 g dietary fiber, 4 mg cholesterol, 528 mg sodium

Italian Minestrone

    1 tablespoon olive oil

    ⅓ cup finely chopped onions

    ⅓ cup finely chopped celery

    ⅓ cup finely chopped carrots

    1 clove garlic, minced

    4 cups fat-free, reduced-sodium chicken broth

    1 can (14 ounces) chopped tomatoes (with juice)

    1 can (16 ounces) canned chickpeas or red kidney beans, rinsed
and drained

    ¾ cup packed chopped escarole or spinach

    ¼ cup uncooked orzo pasta

    1 cup sliced (½" pieces) green beans

    ½ cup finely chopped zucchini

    2 tablespoons chopped fresh basil

In a medium saucepan over medium heat, warm the oil. Add the onions, celery, and carrots; sauté for 5 minutes, or just until softened. Add the garlic and sauté for 1 minute.

Add the broth, tomatoes (with juice), chickpeas or kidney beans, escarole or spinach, and orzo. Bring to a boil over high heat. Reduce the heat to medium and simmer for 10 minutes.

Add the green beans and zucchini. Cover and simmer for 5 minutes, or until the beans are tender. Stir in the basil and cook for 1 minute more.

Makes 4 servings

Per serving: 252 calories, 7.8 g fat (27% of calories), 12.9 g protein, 34.9 g carbohydrates, 7.9 g dietary fiber, 2 mg cholesterol, 629 mg sodium

NOTE:

• Orzo is a type of small pasta that resembles grains of rice. It may be replaced with ¾ cup uncooked small shell pasta.

Split Pea Soup

1 cup dried green split peas, sorted and rinsed

4 cups fat-free chicken broth

1 small onion, finely chopped

1 rib celery, chopped

1 small carrot, finely chopped

¼ teaspoon dried thyme

1 bay leaf

2 teaspoons reduced-sodium soy sauce

2 teaspoons chopped fresh dill

In a large saucepan over high heat, bring the split peas and broth to a boil. Reduce the heat to medium-low, cover, and simmer for 45 minutes, stirring occasionally.

Add the onions, celery, carrots, thyme, bay leaf, and soy sauce. Return to a boil over medium-high heat, then reduce the heat to medium-low. Cover and simmer for 45 minutes, stirring occasionally. Add the dill and cook for another 5 minutes. Remove and discard the bay leaf before serving.

Makes 4 servings

Per serving: 210 calories, 0.7 g fat (3% of calories), 17.5 g protein, 35.2 g carbohydrates, 3 g dietary fiber, 0 mg cholesterol, 447 mg sodium

NOTE:

• Garnish with a swirl of fat-free plain yogurt and a sprinkling of chopped fresh dill.

VARIATION:

• *Split Pea Soup with Ham:* Add ⅓ cup fully cooked chopped lean ham along with the vegetables. Or use the same amount of turkey ham and add 2 drops liquid smoke (available in the condiment section of most supermarkets). Omit the chopped fresh dill.

Tomato Soup

1 tablespoon olive oil

⅓ cup finely chopped onions

¼ cup finely chopped celery

¼ cup finely chopped carrots

1 clove garlic, minced

3 large tomatoes, peeled, seeded, and finely chopped

1 bay leaf

2 tablespoons chopped fresh parsley

2 teaspoons chopped fresh basil

1 teaspoon chopped fresh thyme or ½ teaspoon dried

1 teaspoon chopped fresh marjoram or ½ teaspoon dried

3 cups fat-free chicken broth or reduced-sodium tomato juice

¼ teaspoon ground black pepper

In a large saucepan over medium heat, warm the oil. Add the onions, celery, carrots and garlic and sauté for 5 minutes, or until the onions are soft. Add the tomatoes, bay leaf, parsley, basil, thyme, and marjoram. Cover and cook over low heat for 10 to 15 minutes, or until the mixture is soft and thick.

Gradually stir in the broth or tomato juice and bring to a boil. Reduce the heat to low, cover, and simmer gently for 15 to 20 minutes, or until the vegetables are soft. Stir in the pepper. Remove and discard the bay leaf.

Makes 4 servings

Per serving: 79 calories, 3.8 g fat (40% of calories), 4.7 g protein, 7.9 g carbohydrates, 1.8 g dietary fiber, 0 mg cholesterol, 271 mg sodium

Cobb Salad with Grilled Chicken

Dressing

　　6 tablespoons tomato juice

　　1½ tablespoons red wine vinegar

　　2 teaspoons olive oil

　　½ teaspoon minced garlic

　　½ teaspoon Worcestershire sauce

Salad

　　4 boneless, skinless chicken breast halves

　　4 cups torn mixed lettuce

　　1 cucumber, thinly sliced

　　⅓ cup finely chopped turkey bacon, cooked until crisp

　　2 tomatoes, cut into wedges

　　1½ tablespoons crumbled blue cheese (optional)

To make the dressing: In a small bowl, whisk together the tomato juice, vinegar, oil, garlic, and Worcestershire sauce.

To make the salad: Place the chicken in a glass baking dish and pour half of the dressing over it, reserving the remaining dressing. Cover the dish and marinate the chicken in the refrigerator for 30 minutes.

Remove the chicken and discard any remaining marinade. Grill or broil the chicken for 5 to 8 minutes on each side, or until cooked through (test with a sharp knife). Slice into strips and set aside.

Toss the lettuce and cucumbers with the remaining dressing and place on a platter. Sprinkle with the turkey bacon, arrange the tomatoes around the edge, and garnish with the avocados and blue cheese (if using). Place the chicken in the center of the salad.

Makes 4 servings

Per serving: 194 calories, 8 g fat (36% of calories), 24 g protein, 8.3 g carbohydrates, 1.7 g dietary fiber, 61 mg cholesterol, 359 mg sodium

237

Karla's Spinach Salad

1 pound fresh spinach

8 ounces mushrooms, sliced

2 scallions, thinly sliced

¼ cup crumbled feta cheese

1 clementine or tangerine, segments cut into halves or thirds

2 tablespoons dried cranberries

2 tablespoons walnuts, chopped

1 teaspoon olive oil

1 tablespoon orange juice

3 tablespoons red wine vinegar

1½ teaspoons Dijon mustard

Salt and freshly ground black pepper

In a large bowl, combine the spinach, mushrooms, scallions, cheese, clementine or tangerine, cranberries, and walnuts.

In a small bowl, whisk together the olive oil, orange juice, vinegar, mustard, and salt and pepper to taste.

Pour the dressing over the salad and mix well.

Makes 5 servings

Per serving: 121 calories, 5 g fat (37% of calories), 6 g protein, 13 g carbohydrates, 4 g dietary fiber, 10 mg cholesterol

Macaroni Salad

2 cups cooked elbow macaroni or other tube pasta

1½ tablespoons lemon juice

1 teaspoon canola oil

¾ cup chopped celery

½ cup chopped fresh parsley

½ cup peeled and shredded carrots

½ cup chopped pimiento-stuffed green olives

⅓ cup fat-free sour cream or fat-free plain yogurt

⅓ cup reduced-fat mayonnaise

⅛ teaspoon ground black pepper

⅛ teaspoon paprika

In a medium bowl, combine the macaroni, lemon juice, oil, celery, parsley, carrots, olives, sour cream or yogurt, mayonnaise, and pepper. Cover and refrigerate for 1 hour to allow the flavors to blend. Sprinkle with the paprika before serving.

Makes 4 servings

Per serving: 147 calories, 3.9 g fat (24% of calories), 4.6 g protein, 24.3 g carbohydrates, 2.5 g dietary fiber, 0 mg cholesterol, 736 mg sodium

NOTES:

- For a bit more crunch, add ½ cup chopped green bell peppers.
- Add 2 teaspoons chopped onions or 1 tablespoon chopped fresh chives.

Rich and Creamy Coleslaw

    12 ounces green cabbage, finely shredded
    12 ounces red cabbage, finely shredded
     2 medium carrots, coarsely grated
    ½ cup chopped scallions
    ½ cup fat-free plain yogurt
    ¼ cup fat-free sour cream
     2 tablespoons chopped fresh chives
     1 tablespoon cider vinegar
     2 teaspoons pickle relish
     1 teaspoon honey
    ¼ teaspoon Dijon mustard
    ¼ teaspoon dill, celery, or caraway seeds
    ¼ teaspoon ground black pepper
       Pinch of paprika

In a large bowl, combine the green cabbage, red cabbage, carrots, and scallions.

In a small bowl, whisk together the yogurt, sour cream, chives, vinegar, relish, honey, mustard, dill or celery or caraway seeds, and pepper. Add to the cabbage mixture and toss until well-combined. Cover and refrigerate for at least 1 hour before serving. Just before serving, sprinkle with the paprika.

Makes 4 servings

Per serving: 95 calories, 0.9 g fat (5% of calories), 5.4 g protein, 20.3 g carbohydrates, 4.3 g dietary fiber, 0.5 mg cholesterol, 100 mg sodium

NOTE:

* For extra sweetness and crunch, add ½ cup chopped red bell peppers. Or give the salad a more tangy flavor with ½ cup thinly sliced radishes.

Roasted-Vegetable Salad

1½ pounds small red potatoes, quartered

12 ounces green beans, cut into 1" pieces

2 red bell peppers, thinly sliced

1 red onion, thinly sliced crosswise and separated into rings

½ cup fat-free chicken broth

2 cloves garlic

2 tablespoons red wine vinegar

1½ tablespoons olive oil

1 teaspoon crushed dried rosemary

¼ teaspoon ground black pepper

8 kalamata olives, pitted and sliced

1–2 tablespoons lemon juice

Preheat the oven to 425°.

Coat a 9" × 13" baking dish with cooking spray. Add the potatoes, beans, red peppers, onions, broth, and garlic. Mix well. Roast, stirring every 10 minutes, for 20 to 30 minutes, or until the vegetables are tender. Set aside.

Transfer the garlic to a small bowl and mash. Whisk in the vinegar, oil, rosemary, and black pepper.

Place the vegetables in a large bowl. Add the dressing and olives. Toss to mix well. Sprinkle with the lemon juice just before serving. Serve warm or chilled.

Makes 4 servings

Per serving: 274 calories, 6.9 g fat (21% of calories), 7.2 g protein, 51 g carbohydrates, 3.1 g dietary fiber, 0 mg cholesterol, 215 mg sodium

NOTE:
- The red potatoes can be replaced with peeled and thickly sliced sweet potatoes.

Spinach and Mandarin Orange Salad

Salad

    8 cups torn spinach leaves

    1 red onion, thinly sliced and separated into rings

    ½ cup canned mandarin orange segments, drained

    2 tablespoons toasted sliced almonds

Dressing

    2 tablespoons Dijon mustard

    1 tablespoon honey

    1 tablespoon lemon juice

    1 tablespoon orange juice

To make the salad: In a large bowl, combine the spinach, onions, oranges, and almonds.

To make the dressing: In a small bowl, whisk together the mustard, honey, lemon juice, and orange juice. Pour the dressing over the salad and toss gently to combine.

Makes 4 servings

Per serving: 98 calories, 2.8 g fat (23% of calories), 5.1 g protein, 16.5 g carbohydrates, 4.1 g dietary fiber, 0 mg cholesterol, 192 mg sodium

NOTE:

    • In a pinch, use fat-free honey-mustard dressing.

Three-Bean Picnic Salad

1¼ cups halved green beans

⅔ cup canned chickpeas, rinsed and drained

⅔ cup cooked or canned kidney beans, rinsed and drained

1 medium tomato, seeded and finely chopped

1 tablespoon olive oil

1½ tablespoons Dijon mustard

1½ tablespoons water

1 tablespoon chopped fresh basil

1 teaspoon honey

⅛ teaspoon ground black pepper

2 tablespoons snipped fresh chives

Steam the green beans until crisp-tender, about 5 minutes. Place in a large bowl. Add the chickpeas, kidney beans, and tomatoes. Mix well.

In a food processor or blender, combine the oil, mustard, water, basil, honey, and pepper. Process until smooth. Pour over the salad, sprinkle with the chives, and toss well. Let stand for 20 minutes before serving.

Makes 4 servings

Per serving: 158 calories, 4.9 g fat (27% of calories), 7.4 g protein, 23.3 g carbohydrates, 2.6 g dietary fiber, 0 mg cholesterol, 84 mg sodium

NOTES:

- Use almost any combination of beans. Try fresh limas or wax beans in place of the green beans. Replace the chickpeas or kidney beans with fava, pinto, black, cranberry, or anasazi beans.

- Serve in colorful lettuce cups such as radicchio or Boston lettuce and garnish with chopped fresh basil.

- For a creamier dressing, replace the water with fat-free plain yogurt.

Tricolor Pasta and Spinach Salad

4 cups cooked tricolor rotini

2 cups torn spinach

½ cup chopped scallions

2 tablespoons lemon juice

1 tablespoon red wine vinegar

1 teaspoon olive oil

1 teaspoon Dijon mustard

1 clove garlic, minced

1 tablespoon chopped fresh basil

In a large bowl, combine the pasta, spinach, and scallions.

In a small bowl, whisk the lemon juice, vinegar, oil, mustard, garlic, and basil. Pour the dressing over the salad and toss well to combine.

Makes 4 servings

Per serving: 195 calories, 1.5 g fat (7% of calories), 7.2 g protein, 38.4 g carbohydrates, 6.7 g dietary fiber, 0 mg cholesterol, 47 mg sodium

NOTES:

- To prevent pasta destined for salads from getting soggy, don't over-cook it (it should still be slightly chewy in the center). Drain and run it under cold water to stop the cooking process. Toss with dressing to prevent the pasta from sticking together.

- If you prefer spinach on the softer side, blanch it in boiling water for 30 seconds, plunge it into ice water to stop the cooking process, and coarsely chop before using.

- In a pinch, replace the lemon juice, vinegar, and olive oil with ¼ cup fat-free Italian dressing.

Tuna Salad

3 cans (6 ounces each) drained and flaked water-packed tuna

1 small onion, chopped

½ rib celery, chopped

½ teaspoon lemon juice

1½ tablespoons chopped fresh parsley

⅓ cup fat-free plain yogurt

⅓ cup reduced-calorie mayonnaise

In a medium bowl, combine the tuna, onions, celery, lemon juice, parsley, yogurt, and mayonnaise. Cover and refrigerate for 1 hour to allow the flavors to blend.

Makes 4 servings

Per serving: 139 calories, 5.9 g fat (39% of calories), 15.8 g protein, 4.8 g carbohydrates, 0.4 g dietary fiber, 24 mg cholesterol, 232 mg sodium

VARIATIONS:

- *Seafood Salad:* Replace the tuna with other seafood such as shrimp, crabmeat, or salmon.
- *Tangy Tuna Salad:* Replace half of the parsley with chopped fresh chives.

Waldorf Salad

1 cup thinly sliced apples

¼ cup thinly sliced celery

½ cup seedless green grapes

1½ tablespoons apple juice

1 tablespoon lemon juice

1 teaspoon extra-virgin olive oil

½ teaspoon Dijon mustard

3 cups torn romaine lettuce

1 head Belgian endive, leaves separated

1 tablespoon coarsely chopped toasted walnuts (see note)

In a medium bowl, combine the apples, celery, and grapes.

In a small bowl, combine the apple juice, lemon juice, oil, and mustard; mix well. Toss the apple mixture with 1½ tablespoons of the dressing.

Place the romaine on a serving platter and arrange the endive leaves in a wheel on top of the romaine. Drizzle the greens with the remaining dressing. Place the apple mixture in the center of the platter and top with the walnuts.

Makes 4 servings

Per serving: 71 calories, 2.7 g fat (31% of calories), 1.9 g protein, 11.6 g carbohydrates, 2.7 g dietary fiber, 0 mg cholesterol, 27 mg sodium

NOTES:

- To toast walnuts, place them in dry skillet over medium heat. Toast the nuts, shaking the pan often, for 3 to 5 minutes, or until fragrant and golden.

- For a more fruity salad, add ½ cup blueberries.

- Sprinkle the top of the salad with 1½ tablespoons crumbled blue cheese.

Apple-Walnut Muffins

2 cups whole wheat flour

½ cup sugar

2 teaspoons baking powder

½ teaspoon baking soda

½ teaspoon salt

1 teaspoon ground cinnamon

¼ cup chopped walnuts

2 large Granny Smith apples, peeled and grated

1 large egg

1 teaspoon vanilla extract

1 cup 1% milk

Preheat the oven to 350°. Coat a 12-cup muffin pan with cooking spray.

In a medium bowl, combine the flour, sugar, baking powder, baking soda, salt, cinnamon, and walnuts.

In a large bowl, combine the apples, eggs, vanilla, and milk.

Add the dry ingredients and blend well.

Divide the batter equally among the prepared muffin cups, filling them three-quarters full. Bake for 15 minutes, or until the muffin tops are lightly browned and a wooden pick inserted in the center comes out clean.

Makes 12

Per muffin: 155 calories, 4 g fat (23% of calories), 4 g protein, 28 g carbohydrates, 3 g dietary fiber, 19 g cholesterol

Banana Bread

   1¾ cups whole wheat flour

   ¾ cup sugar

   2 teaspoons baking powder

   ½ teaspoon baking soda

   ½ teaspoon salt

   ¼ cup walnuts, chopped

   3 ripe bananas

   2 large eggs

   1 teaspoon vanilla extract

Preheat the oven to 325°. Lightly coat an 8½" × 4½" loaf pan with cooking spray.

In a medium bowl, combine the flour, sugar, baking powder, baking soda, salt, and walnuts.

In a large bowl, mash the bananas with a fork. Add the eggs and vanilla and stir to combine.

Add the dry ingredients and blend well.

Pour the batter into the prepared pan and bake for 1 hour, or until a wooden pick inserted in the center comes out clean.

Makes 1 loaf; 10 slices

Per slice: 203 calories, 3 g fat (13% of calories), 5 g protein, 39 g carbohydrates, 4 g dietary fiber, 43 mg cholesterol

Basic Scones

> 1 cup + 2 tablespoons all-purpose flour
>
> 1 cup cake flour
>
> ½ cup rolled oats
>
> 2 tablespoons sugar
>
> 2½ teaspoons baking powder
>
> ¼ teaspoon salt
>
> 3 tablespoons nondiet tub-style margarine or butter
>
> ½ cup fat-free milk
>
> 2 egg whites

Preheat the oven to 425°. Coat a nonstick baking sheet with cooking spray.

In a medium bowl, combine the all-purpose flour, cake flour, oats, sugar, baking powder, and salt; set aside.

Using 2 table knives or a pastry blender, cut the margarine into the flour mixture until coarse crumbs form. Using a fork, stir in the milk and egg whites until a dough forms.

Turn the dough out onto a lightly floured surface and gently knead for 1 minute. Using a floured rolling pin, gently roll the dough into a ½"-thick rectangle, or pat into shape using your hands. Using a 2" biscuit cutter, cut the dough into rounds. Reroll as necessary to cut 12 scones.

Place the scones on the prepared baking sheet. Lightly coat the top of the scones with cooking spray. Bake for 12 to 15 minutes, or until the bottoms of the scones are lightly browned and the tops are golden.

Makes 12

Per scone: 129 calories, 3.3 g fat (23% of calories), 3.5 g protein, 21.1 g carbohydrates, 0.8 g dietary fiber, 0.2 mg cholesterol, 166 mg sodium

Bran Muffins

½ cup all-purpose flour

½ cup whole wheat flour

1 tablespoon baking powder

¼ teaspoon salt

¼ teaspoon cinnamon

1 cup fat-free milk

2 tablespoons canola oil

2 tablespoons honey

3 egg whites

1 cup all-bran cereal

Preheat the oven to 400°. Spray a 12-cup nonstick muffin pan with cooking spray or line the cups with paper liners.

In a medium bowl, combine the all-purpose flour, whole wheat flour, baking powder, salt, and cinnamon; set aside.

In a small bowl, stir together the milk, oil, honey, and egg whites. Stir in the cereal and let stand for 10 minutes. Gently stir the milk mixture into the flour mixture just until a lumpy batter forms.

Divide the batter equally among the prepared muffin cups, filling them two-thirds full. Bake for 20 to 25 minutes, or until the muffin tops are lightly browned and a wooden pick inserted in the center comes out clean.

Cool in the pan on a rack for 10 minutes. Remove from the pan and serve warm or cool completely.

Makes 12

Per muffin: 97 calories, 2.6 g fat (22% of calories), 3.8 g protein, 17.1 g carbohydrates, 2.9 g dietary fiber, 0.3 mg cholesterol, 231 mg sodium

Corn Muffins

1 cup all-purpose flour

1 cup cornmeal

2 tablespoons sugar

2½ teaspoons baking powder

¼ teaspoon baking soda

¼ teaspoon salt

2 tablespoons canola oil

2 tablespoons unsweetened applesauce

2 egg whites, lightly beaten

1 cup buttermilk

Preheat the oven to 400°. Spray a 12-cup nonstick muffin pan with cooking spray or line the cups with paper liners.

In a medium bowl, combine the flour, cornmeal, sugar, baking powder, baking soda, and salt; set aside. Using a fork, stir in the oil, applesauce, and egg whites until well-distributed. Stir in the buttermilk just until a lumpy batter forms.

Divide the batter evenly among the prepared muffin cups, filling them two-thirds full. Bake for 20 minutes, or until the muffin tops are lightly browned and a wooden pick inserted in the center comes out clean.

Cool in the pan on a rack for 10 minutes. Remove from the pan and serve warm or cool completely.

Makes 12

Per muffin: 116 calories, 2.9 g fat (23% of calories), 3.2 g protein, 19.4 g carbohydrates, 1.9 g dietary fiber, 1 mg cholesterol, 174 mg sodium

Cinnamon Buns with Coffee Glaze

Dough

2 packages (¼ ounce each) active dry yeast

½ cup warm water (105°–115°)

1 cup fat-free milk, scalded and cooled to lukewarm

1 large egg, beaten

¼ cup sugar

1 teaspoon salt

3½–4 cups all-purpose flour

Filling

1 cup packed brown sugar

2 teaspoons cinnamon

3 tablespoons softened butter

Glaze

1 cup confectioners' sugar

Pinch of salt

1 teaspoon vanilla extract

1–3 teaspoons strong hot coffee

To make the dough: In a large bowl, dissolve the yeast in the water. Let stand for 5 minutes, or until the yeast is foamy. Stir in the milk, egg, sugar, and salt. Stir in 2 cups of the flour and beat until the batter is smooth and elastic. Gradually stir in enough of the remaining flour to make a dough that forms an irregular ball. Let the dough rest for 15 minutes.

Turn the dough out onto a lightly floured surface and knead, adding flour as necessary, until the dough is smooth and satiny.

Coat a clean large bowl with cooking spray. Place the dough in the bowl, cover with a damp cloth, and let rise for 1 hour, or until doubled in bulk.

To make the filling: Coat a 9" × 13" nonstick baking pan with cooking spray and set aside. In a small bowl, combine the brown sugar and cinnamon and set aside.

Roll the dough out to make a 24" × 14" rectangle. Spread the softened butter over the dough. Sprinkle with the brown-sugar mixture. Starting with the long end, tightly roll the dough. When completely rolled, pinch the edges to seal. Cut into 1" slices and place the slices, cut side down, close together in the prepared pan. Let rise for 45 minutes, or until puffy and almost doubled in bulk.

Preheat the oven to 350°. Bake the buns for 25 to 30 minutes, or until golden.

To make the glaze: In a small bowl, mix the confectioners' sugar, salt, and vanilla. Stir in the coffee, 1 teaspoon at a time, until the mixture is smooth and pourable. Drizzle over the warm rolls.

Makes 24

Per bun: 149 calories, 1.9 g fat (11% of calories), 2.8 g protein, 30.4 g carbohydrates, 0.7 g dietary fiber, 13 mg cholesterol, 114 mg sodium

Herb Dinner Rolls

½ cup water

½ cup + 1 tablespoon fat-free milk

1 package (¼ ounce) quick-rising yeast

1 tablespoon olive oil

1 teaspoon honey

   About 1¾ cups unbleached flour, divided

½ cup whole wheat flour

½ teaspoon dried thyme

½ teaspoon dried rosemary, crumbled

½ teaspoon salt

¼ teaspoon ground black pepper

In a small microwaveable bowl, combine the water and ½ cup of the milk. Microwave on high power for 30 seconds, or until lukewarm. Mix in the yeast, oil, and honey. Let stand for 5 minutes, or until the yeast is foamy.

In a food processor, combine the unbleached flour, whole wheat flour, thyme, rosemary, salt, and pepper. Process briefly to mix well. With the machine running, pour in the yeast mixture through the feed tube. Process for about 1 minute, or until the mixture forms a ball of dough that sits on top of the blade.

Turn the dough out onto a lightly floured surface. Knead for 5 minutes, or until the dough is smooth. (If necessary, add a little more flour to keep the dough from sticking.)

Coat a clean large bowl with cooking spray. Place the dough in the prepared bowl. Cover with a damp cloth and let rise in a warm place for 30 minutes, or until doubled in bulk.

Gently deflate the dough with your fist and turn out onto a lightly floured surface. Knead for 1 minute. Form into a rope about 18" long. Cut into 12 equal pieces. Form each piece into a ball.

Preheat the oven to 400°. Coat a nonstick baking sheet with cooking spray. Place the balls on the sheet, leaving about 2" between them. Cover with a damp towel and let rise in a warm, draft-free place for 15 minutes, or until doubled in bulk. Uncover and lightly brush the balls with the remaining 1 tablespoon milk.

Bake for 15 to 20 minutes, or until the rolls are lightly browned.

Makes 12

Per roll: 101 calories, 1.4 g fat (13% of calories), 3.2 g protein, 18.9 g carbohydrates, 1.3 g dietary fiber, 0.2 mg cholesterol, 95 mg sodium

NOTE:

- To save time, let the dough rise in the microwave. Microwave on low power for 5 minutes. (Do not use a higher power, because the heat may kill the yeast.) Give the bowl a quarter-turn, then microwave on low power for another 5 minutes. If the dough has not doubled in bulk, microwave on low power for another 5 minutes.

French Toast

¾ cup fat-free milk

¾ cup liquid egg substitute

1 teaspoon canola oil

½ teaspoon vanilla extract

¼ teaspoon ground cinnamon

8 slices oat-bran or whole wheat bread

In a 9" × 13" nonstick baking dish, combine the milk, egg substitute, oil, vanilla, and cinnamon. Add the bread in a single layer and soak until most of the liquid is absorbed. Using a spatula, turn the bread slices to coat both sides with the egg mixture.

Coat a griddle or large nonstick skillet with cooking spray. Place over medium heat until hot. Using a spatula, transfer the bread slices to the pan, working in batches if necessary. Brown on both sides.

Makes 4 servings

Per serving: 190 calories, 3.8 g fat (18% of calories), 11.6 g protein, 27 g carbohydrates, 0 g dietary fiber, 1 mg cholesterol, 345 mg sodium

Whole Wheat Bread

2 packages (¼ ounce each) active dry yeast

2½ cups warm water (105°–115°)

¼ cup honey

2 teaspoons salt

1 tablespoon canola oil

6–6½ cups whole wheat bread flour

In a large bowl, dissolve the yeast in the water. Stir in the honey and let stand for 5 minutes, or until the yeast is foamy. Stir in the salt, oil, and 2 cups of the flour. Beat until smooth. Stir in enough of the remaining flour to make a dough that comes together in an irregular ball. Cover with a damp cloth and let the dough rest for 15 minutes.

Turn the dough out onto a lightly floured surface and knead for 10 to 15 minutes, or until the dough is smooth and elastic.

Coat a clean large bowl with cooking spray. Place the dough in the bowl, cover with a damp towel, and let rise in a warm place for 35 to 45 minutes, or until the dough is light and doubled in bulk.

Coat two 9" × 5" or 8" × 4" nonstick loaf pans with cooking spray. Gently deflate the dough with your fist and knead to eliminate air bubbles. Divide the dough into 2 equal pieces and shape into oblong loaves. Place in the prepared pans, cover with a damp cloth, and let rise in a warm place for 40 to 45 minutes, or until the dough is light and almost doubled in bulk.

Preheat the oven to 375°. Bake the loaves for 30 minutes. Reduce the oven temperature to 350° and bake for 10 to 15 minutes longer, or until a wooden pick inserted in the center comes out clean. Immediately remove from the pans and cool on a rack.

Makes 2 loaves; 16 slices each

Per slice: 89 calories, 0.8 g fat (8% of calories), 3.2 g protein, 18.5 g carbohydrates, 3 g dietary fiber, 0 mg cholesterol, 135 mg sodium

Milwaukee Pumpernickel Bread

1 cup mashed potatoes

½ cup rolled oats

1 cup rye flour

½ cup stone-ground cornmeal

⅓ cup wheat germ

⅓ cup dark molasses

2 teaspoons salt

2 cups boiling water

1 teaspoon instant coffee powder

½ cup warm water (105°–115°)

2 packages (¼ ounce each) active dry yeast

2 cups whole wheat flour

2½–3 cups bread flour

In a large bowl, combine the potatoes, oats, rye flour, cornmeal, wheat germ, molasses, salt, boiling water, and coffee powder. Stir well and set aside until the mixture has cooled to 105° to 115°.

Place the warm water in a small bowl. Sprinkle with the yeast and set aside for 2 minutes, or until the yeast is foamy. Stir the yeast mixture into the cooled potato mixture. Stir in the whole wheat flour and beat well. Add the bread flour gradually to make a stiff dough that clears the edge of the bowl. Let the dough rest for 15 minutes.

Turn the dough out onto a lightly floured surface and knead for 10 minutes, or until the dough is smooth and free of any dry flour lumps. (The dough will not be as springy as white-flour dough, but it should feel well-mixed. It may be slightly sticky, but do not add too much additional flour.)

Coat a clean large bowl with cooking spray. Place the dough in the bowl and cover with a damp cloth. Let rise in a warm place for 1 to 1½ hours, or until doubled in bulk.

Turn the dough out onto a surface lightly coated with cooking spray and divide into 2 equal pieces. Shape each piece into an oblong loaf about 12" long.

Coat a nonstick baking sheet with cooking spray. Place the loaves on the prepared baking sheet, cover with a damp cloth, and let rise for 45 to 60 minutes, or until puffy.

Preheat the oven to 375°. Bake the loaves for 30 to 40 minutes, or until deep golden brown. Cool on a rack.

Makes 2 loaves; 22 slices each.

Per slice: 76 calories, 0.4 g fat (5% of calories), 2.6 g protein, 16 g carbohydrates, 1.5 g dietary fiber, 0 mg cholesterol, 115 mg sodium

NOTES:

- For a less sweet pumpernickel, reduce the molasses to ¼ cup.
- For best results, wait until the second day to cut this loaf into thin slices.

Sourdough Bread

Sourdough Starter

    1 package (¼ ounce) active dry yeast

    1 teaspoon sugar

1–1½ cups warm water (105°–115°)

    2 cups all-purpose flour

Bread Dough

    1 cup warm water (105°–115°)

    2 teaspoons salt

4½–5 cups bread flour

To make the sourdough starter: In a large plastic bowl with a tight-fitting lid, combine the yeast, sugar, water, and flour. Loosely cover and let stand in a warm place for 5 days, stirring at least once a day. When the starter is ready for use, it will be bubbly and may have a layer of yellow liquid on top. Stir well before using.

To make the bread dough: Add the warm water, salt, and 1 cup of the flour to the starter and stir. Gradually stir in enough of the remaining flour to make a very stiff dough. Turn the dough out onto a lightly floured surface and knead until smooth and elastic, adding flour as needed. (You may also turn the dough into the bowl of a heavy-duty mixer with a dough hook and knead for 8 to 10 minutes, or until smooth and elastic.)

Coat a clean large bowl with cooking spray. Place the dough in the bowl, cover with a damp towel, and let rise in a warm place for 2 hours, or until doubled in bulk.

At this point, you may use all of the dough to make 1 loaf of bread or remove some of the dough to repeat the starter process (so you can make more bread in the future). To repeat the starter process, remove 1 cup of the risen dough and place it in the plastic starter bowl. Pour 1½ cups warm water over the starter dough. Stir in 1 cup flour. Cover and let stand at room temperature until doubled in bulk. Then, refrigerate the starter until you are ready to bake again (see note).

Shape the remaining bread dough into a round loaf about 2½" thick. Coat a nonstick baking sheet with cooking spray. Place the loaf on the sheet. Loosely cover with a damp cloth and let rise for 1 to 2 hours, or until doubled in bulk.

Preheat the oven to 400°. With a sharp knife, make three ¼"-deep slits on the top of the loaf. Bake for 20 to 25 minutes, or until golden and crusty. Remove the bread from the baking sheet and cool on a rack.

Makes 1 large loaf; 24 slices

Per slice: 106 calories, 0.3 g fat (2% of calories), 3.1 g protein, 22.2 g carbohydrates, 0.9 g dietary fiber, 0 mg cholesterol, 178 mg sodium

NOTES:

- It takes 5 days to develop the sourdough flavor in this starter. Once the starter is made, you can keep making bread from it by repeating the directions under "to make the bread dough."

- If you don't plan to make bread again within a week, you can refrigerate the starter indefinitely by refreshing it once a week. To do this, remove 1 cup of the starter. Into the remaining starter, stir 1½ cups warm water and 1 cup flour. Cover and let stand at room temperature until doubled in bulk. Refrigerate and repeat until you are ready to make bread.

VARIATIONS:

- *Sourdough Hard Rolls:* Divide the risen dough into 12 equal pieces. Lightly coat a nonstick baking sheet with cooking spray. Place the dough pieces on the baking sheet. Cover with a damp cloth and let rise in a warm place for 1 to 2 hours, or until doubled in bulk. Bake at 400° for 12 to 15 minutes, or until golden.

- *Sourdough Breadsticks:* Divide the risen dough in half. Divide each half into 32 equal pieces. Shape each piece into an 8"-long breadstick. Lightly coat a nonstick baking sheet with cooking spray. Place the dough pieces on the baking sheet. Lightly brush the breadsticks with beaten egg white and sprinkle with sesame seeds. Cover with a damp cloth and let rise in a warm place for 30 minutes, or until doubled in bulk. Bake at 400° for 15 minutes, or until golden. Makes 64.

Baked Ziti

8 ounces ziti

8 ounces low-fat Italian turkey sausage, casings removed

1 jar (27½ ounces) reduced-sodium tomato sauce

1½ cups shredded fat-free mozzarella cheese

1 tablespoon grated Parmesan cheese

2 tablespoons chopped fresh parsley

Preheat the oven to 350°. Coat a shallow 2½-quart nonstick baking dish with cooking spray and set aside.

In a large pot of boiling water, cook the ziti according to the package directions.

Meanwhile, in a large nonstick skillet coated with cooking spray, cook and stir the sausage for 5 to 7 minutes, or until broken into small pieces and no longer pink.

Drain the ziti and place in a large bowl. Add the sausage, tomato sauce, and 1 cup of the mozzarella and mix well. Spoon into the prepared baking dish.

Cover with foil and bake for 30 minutes. Uncover and sprinkle with the Parmesan and the remaining ½ cup mozzarella. Bake for 6 to 8 minutes, or until the cheese melts. Sprinkle with the parsley before serving.

Makes 4 servings

Per serving: 457 calories, 5.5 g fat (11% of calories), 36.5 g protein, 63 g carbohydrates, 2.9 g dietary fiber, 37 mg cholesterol, 864 mg sodium

NOTES:

- This dish can be assembled a day ahead and refrigerated, then baked when needed. Increase the initial baking time from 30 to 35 minutes.

- You may replace the ziti with other short tube pasta such as penne or rigatoni.

Bow Ties with Greens and Beans

12 ounces bow-tie noodles

1 teaspoon olive oil

2 cups broccoli florets

1 red onion, thinly sliced and separated into rings

2 cloves garlic, minced

1 tablespoon all-purpose flour

2 cups fat-free, reduced-sodium chicken broth or vegetable broth

1 bunch (about 1 pound) escarole, chopped into 1" pieces

1 can (16 ounces) chickpeas, rinsed and drained

2 tablespoons grated Parmesan cheese

2 teaspoons lemon juice

In a large pot of boiling water, cook the bow ties according to the package directions.

Meanwhile, in a large nonstick skillet over medium heat, warm the oil. Add the broccoli, onions, and garlic and cook, stirring frequently, for 4 minutes, or until the broccoli is bright green and crisp-tender. Transfer the broccoli mixture to a small bowl.

Sprinkle the flour into the skillet. Cook and stir for 1 minute. Gradually whisk in the broth until blended and smooth.

Add the broccoli mixture, escarole, chickpeas, Parmesan, and lemon juice and bring to a boil. Reduce the heat to low, cover, and simmer for 5 to 7 minutes, or until the vegetables are tender and the sauce thickens slightly. Drain the pasta and place in a large serving bowl. Add the sauce and toss to mix well.

Makes 4 servings

Per serving: 536 calories, 5.6 g fat (9% of calories), 24.4 g protein, 99.2 g carbohydrates, 12.1 g dietary fiber, 0 mg cholesterol, 581 mg sodium

Cavatelli with Broccoli

12 ounces cavatelli

2 cups broccoli florets

1 tablespoon olive oil

½ cup finely chopped red onions

2 cloves garlic, minced

½ cup fat-free, reduced-sodium chicken broth

2 teaspoons balsamic vinegar

½ cup finely chopped roasted red peppers

2 tablespoons grated Parmesan cheese

¼ teaspoon ground black pepper

2 tablespoons chopped fresh basil (optional)

In a large pot of boiling water, cook the cavatelli according to the package directions. Add the broccoli and cook for 3 to 4 minutes, or until the pasta is tender and the broccoli is bright green.

Meanwhile, in a large nonstick skillet over medium heat, warm the oil. Add the onions and garlic and sauté for 2 to 3 minutes, or until the onions are tender. Stir in the broth and vinegar and bring to a boil. Reduce the heat to low and stir in the red peppers, Parmesan, and black pepper. Cook for 1 to 2 minutes, or until heated through.

Drain the pasta and broccoli and place in a large serving bowl. Add the onion mixture and toss to mix well. Sprinkle with the basil (if using).

Makes 4 servings

Per serving: 413 calories, 5.7 g fat (12% of calories), 16.1 g protein, 75.8 g carbohydrates, 3.9 g dietary fiber, 0 mg cholesterol, 114 mg sodium

NOTES:

- For extra garlic flavor, rub the cut side of a garlic clove around the serving bowl before tossing the pasta and sauce.
- You can replace the cavatelli with bow-tie noodles or medium shells.

Classic Lasagna

12 lasagna noodles

½ cup liquid egg substitute

2 cups fat-free ricotta cheese

2 cups reduced-fat ricotta cheese

¼ cup chopped fresh parsley

4 cups tomato sauce

2 cups shredded reduced-fat mozzarella cheese

Preheat the oven to 375°.

In a large pot of boiling water, cook the noodles according to the package directions. Drain.

Meanwhile, in a large bowl, combine the egg substitute, fat-free ricotta, reduced-fat ricotta, and parsley; set aside.

Spread 1 cup of the tomato sauce in the bottom of a 9" × 13" nonstick baking dish. Place a layer of 4 noodles in the dish. Sprinkle with half of the mozzarella. Spread a layer of the filling over the mozzarella. Spoon on a layer of sauce. Add a layer of 4 noodles, then top with all but ¼ cup of the remaining mozzarella. Spread on the remaining filling. Finish with the remaining 4 noodles and the remaining sauce. Sprinkle with the reserved mozzarella.

Cover loosely with foil. Bake for 30 to 35 minutes, or until the cheese is browned and bubbly and the lasagna is heated through. Let stand for 10 minutes before cutting.

Makes 10 servings

Per serving: 267 calories, 8.7 g fat (29% of calories), 22.6 g protein, 26.2 g carbohydrates, 2.9 g dietary fiber, 28 mg cholesterol, 667 mg sodium

Linguine with White Clam Sauce

4 dozen littleneck clams, scrubbed

4 teaspoons all-purpose flour

2 teaspoons olive oil

3 cloves garlic, minced

3 bay leaves

2 cups fat-free chicken broth

½ cup fat-free evaporated milk

2 teaspoons Dijon mustard

¼ teaspoon dried thyme

8 ounces linguine

Place the clams in a Dutch oven or deep, heavy pot. Add 1" of water and bring to a boil. Reduce the heat to medium, cover, and steam for 6 to 10 minutes, or just until the clams open. With a slotted spoon, remove the clams and discard any that did not open. Let the clams cool, then remove them from their shells. Mince the clams and transfer to a large bowl. Add the flour and toss to coat; set aside.

In a large nonstick skillet over medium heat, warm the oil. Add the garlic and bay leaves and sauté for 4 minutes, or until the garlic begins to brown. Add the broth, milk, mustard, and thyme. Cook, stirring frequently, until the sauce is reduced by about half. Add the reserved clams. Cook and stir for 2 minutes, or until the sauce thickens.

Meanwhile, in a large pot of boiling water, cook the linguine for 8 to 10 minutes, or just until tender. Drain and transfer to a serving bowl.

Remove the bay leaves from the sauce and discard. Toss the pasta with the sauce.

Makes 4 servings

Per serving: 247 calories, 3.8 g fat (14% of calories), 17 g protein, 36.4 g carbohydrates, 0.1 g dietary fiber, 19 mg cholesterol, 241 mg sodium

Macaroni and Cheese

> 6 ounces elbow macaroni (about 1½ cups)
>
> ⅔ cup shredded reduced-fat Cheddar cheese
>
> ½ cup dry-curd cottage cheese
>
> ½ cup fat-free milk
>
> ½ cup liquid egg substitute
>
> ¼ teaspoon hot-pepper sauce
>
> 1 teaspoon Dijon mustard
>
> ¼ cup seasoned dry bread crumbs
>
> ¼ teaspoon paprika
>
> 1 tablespoon grated Parmesan cheese

In a large pot of boiling water, cook the macaroni according to the package directions. Drain.

Preheat the oven to 375°.

Coat a 1-quart nonstick baking dish with cooking spray. Add the macaroni and Cheddar. Toss to combine.

In a food processor or blender, puree the cottage cheese, milk, egg substitute, hot-pepper sauce, and ½ teaspoon of the mustard. Pour over the macaroni and stir to combine.

In a small bowl, mix the bread crumbs with the paprika, Parmesan, and the remaining ½ teaspoon mustard. Sprinkle over the macaroni. Bake for 25 minutes.

Makes 4 servings

Per serving: 321 calories, 7.1 g fat (20% of calories), 22.1 g protein, 40.3 g carbohydrates, 0 g dietary fiber, 23 mg cholesterol, 944 mg sodium

VARIATION:

- *Tomato Macaroni and Cheese:* Gently stir 10 halved cherry tomatoes into the macaroni mixture before adding the cheese sauce. For a tangier taste, add 1 tablespoon chopped onions.

Mediterranean Pasta with Shrimp

1 clove garlic, minced

1 large onion, chopped

2 tablespoons dry sherry or nonalcoholic white wine

2 tablespoons + ⅓ cup fat-free chicken broth

1 can (16 ounces) reduced-sodium stewed tomatoes (with juice)

1 jar (14¾ ounces) water-packed artichoke hearts, drained

5 large pimiento-stuffed green olives, sliced

2 teaspoons dried Italian seasoning

¼ teaspoon ground black pepper

1 pound medium shrimp (40 to 50 shrimp), shelled and deveined

8 ounces fusilli

Coat a large nonstick skillet with cooking spray. Add the garlic, onions, sherry or wine, and 2 tablespoons of the broth. Cook, stirring, over medium heat for 5 mintues, or until the onions are tender.

Add the tomatoes (with juice), artichokes, olives, Italian seasoning, pepper, and the remaining ⅓ cup broth. Add the shrimp and simmer, uncovered, for 3 minutes, or until the shrimp turn pink.

Meanwhile, in a large pot of boiling water, cook the fusilli according to the package directions. Drain. Serve the shrimp mixture over the fusilli.

Makes 4 servings

Per serving: 490 calories, 3.5 g fat (6% of calories), 34.6 g protein, 80 g carbohydrates, 6.8 g dietary fiber, 175 mg cholesterol, 460 mg sodium

> VARIATION:
>
> • *Pasta with Scallops:* Replace the shrimp with 1 pound bay or sea scallops. The slightly smaller bay scallops have a superior flavor. If using bay scallops, reduce the cooking time to 2 to 3 minutes. If using sea scallops, cook for 3 to 6 minutes. Cook the scallops just until done; the interior should still be tender.

Pasta with Creamy Parmesan Sauce

8 ounces fusilli

3 tablespoons dry sherry or nonalcoholic white wine

1 tablespoon water

1 tablespoon nondiet tub-style margarine or butter

1 large onion, finely chopped

1 small clove garlic, minced

2 tablespoons all-purpose flour

½ teaspoon dry mustard

⅛ teaspoon ground black pepper

1¾ cups 1% milk

½ cup grated reduced-fat Parmesan cheese

⅓ cup fat-free sour cream

1 tablespoon chopped fresh parsley

In a large pot of boiling water, cook the fusilli according to the package directions. Drain. Transfer to a large bowl and keep warm.

Meanwhile, in a large nonstick skillet over medium heat, warm the sherry or wine, water, and margarine or butter. Add the onions and garlic. Cook and stir for 7 to 8 minutes, or until the onions are tender. If the liquid begins to evaporate, add a bit more water.

Whisk in the flour, mustard, and pepper. Gradually whisk in the milk. Cook and stir for 4 to 5 minutes, or until the sauce begins to thicken. Reduce the heat to medium-low to prevent the sauce from boiling. Add the Parmesan and stir until melted. Stir in the sour cream and cook over low heat for 1 to 2 minutes.

Toss the fusilli with the sauce. Garnish with the parsley.

Makes 4 servings

Per serving: 403 calories, 8.9 g fat (20% of calories), 18.4 g protein, 59 g carbohydrates, 0.9 dietary fiber, 14 mg cholesterol, 340 mg sodium

Penne with Broccoli and Peppers

8 ounces penne

2 cups broccoli florets

1 tablespoon olive oil

1 red or yellow bell pepper, cut into thin strips

3 large cloves garlic, slivered

½ cup vegetable or fat-free chicken broth

1¼ teaspoons Dijon mustard

½ teaspoon salt (optional)

⅛ teaspoon ground black pepper

2 teaspoons balsamic vinegar

2 tablespoons grated Parmesan cheese (optional)

In a large pot of boiling water, cook the penne according to the package directions. Drain. Transfer to a serving bowl and keep warm.

Meanwhile, in a medium saucepan, cook the broccoli in a small amount of boiling water for 5 minutes, or until bright green and just tender. Drain.

In a large nonstick skillet over medium heat, warm the oil. Add the red or yellow peppers and sauté for 2 minutes. Add the garlic and sauté for 2 minutes.

Stir in the broth and broccoli and cook for 3 minutes. Stir in the mustard, salt (if using), and black pepper.

Toss the penne with the vegetables. Drizzle with the vinegar and toss again. Sprinkle with the Parmesan (if using).

Makes 4 servings

Per serving: 291 calories, 4.9 g fat (15% of calories), 9.9 g protein, 53 g carbohydrates, 2.6 g dietary fiber, 0 mg cholesterol, 45 mg sodium

Stuffed Shells Florentine

2 cups reduced-sodium spaghetti sauce

16 jumbo pasta shells (about 5–6 ounces)

1½ cups reduced-fat ricotta cheese

1 package (10 ounces) frozen chopped spinach, thawed and squeezed dry

½ cup coarsely chopped reduced-sodium stewed tomatoes

¼ cup grated reduced-fat Parmesan cheese

1 tablespoon fat-free milk

1 teaspoon dried basil

⅛ teaspoon ground nutmeg

⅓ cup shredded fat-free mozzarella cheese

Preheat the oven to 350°. Spread 1 cup of the spaghetti sauce in the bottom of a 9" × 13" nonstick baking dish and set aside.

In a large pot of boiling water, cook the shells according to the package directions.

Meanwhile, in a large bowl, combine the ricotta, spinach, tomatoes, Parmesan, milk, basil, nutmeg, and half of the mozzarella.

Drain the shells. Spoon equal amounts of the filling into the shells and place them, filling side up, in the prepared baking dish. Spoon the remaining 1 cup spaghetti sauce over them.

Cover with foil and bake for 40 minutes. Uncover and sprinkle with the remaining mozzarella. Bake for 5 to 10 minutes, or until the cheese melts.

Makes 4 servings

Per serving: 358 calories, 5.8 g fat (15% of calories), 21.8 g protein, 55.1 g carbohydrates, 0.4 g dietary fiber, 12 mg cholesterol, 643 mg sodium

Spaghetti and Meatballs

   1½ slices whole wheat bread, torn into small pieces

     4 ounces ground turkey breast

     4 ounces low-fat turkey sausage, casings removed

     2 tablespoons chopped onions

     2 teaspoons minced garlic

     ½ teaspoon dried basil

     ½ teaspoon dried oregano

       Pinch of ground red pepper

     1 egg white, lightly beaten

     ½ cup fat-free chicken broth

     1 small onion, finely chopped

     2 red bell peppers, finely chopped

     4 large tomatoes, seeded and finely chopped

     ¼ cup tomato sauce

     8 ounces spaghetti

Place the bread in a food processor or blender and process with on/off turns to make fine crumbs. Crumble the turkey breast and turkey sausage into the food processor. Add the chopped onions, garlic, basil, oregano, and ground red pepper and process briefly. Add the egg white and process with on/off turns until well-mixed. Shape the mixture into 1" balls.

Coat a Dutch oven or large nonstick skillet with cooking spray. Place over medium heat, add the meatballs, and brown on all sides. Remove to a platter and set aside.

Add the broth to the pan and scrape up the cooked-on particles of meat with a wooden spoon. Add the finely chopped onions and red peppers. Sauté, stirring frequently, for 5 minutes, or until tender. Add the tomatoes and tomato sauce. Cover and cook for 10 minutes, stirring frequently to prevent scorching. Add the meatballs and cook for 10 minutes more.

Meanwhile, in a large pot of boiling water, cook the spaghetti according to the package directions. Drain and serve with the meatballs and sauce.

Makes 4 servings

Per serving: 460 calories, 7.6 g fat (15% of calories), 25.7 g protein, 74.2 g carbohydrates, 4.4 g dietary fiber, 42 mg cholesterol, 402 mg sodium

NOTE:

- To buy the leanest ground turkey available, look for products made with only turkey breast meat. Many ground turkey products also contain the dark meat and fatty skin.

Vegetable Pasta Sauce

   1 large eggplant, cut into 1" cubes

   2 cloves garlic, chopped

   1 large onion, sliced

   1 large green bell pepper, sliced

   1 large red bell pepper, sliced

   1 small zucchini, cut into ¼"-thick slices

   1 medium yellow squash, cut into ¼"-thick slices

   1 can (28 ounces) crushed tomatoes

   1 can (12 ounces) tomato paste

   ¼ cup chopped fresh Italian parsley

   ½ cup chopped fresh basil

   1 tablespoon dried oregano

      Salt and freshly ground black pepper

   ½ cup grated Parmesan cheese

   1 teaspoon sugar

Line a colander with a paper towel. Place the eggplant in the colander and sprinkle with salt. Let stand for at least 20 minutes.

Coat the bottom of an 8-quart pot with cooking spray. Add the garlic and onion and sauté until transparent.

Add the red peppers and green peppers and cook until soft.

Add the reserved eggplant, the zucchini, yellow squash, tomatoes, tomato paste, parsley, basil, oregano, salt, pepper, and ¼ cup of the Parmesan. Cook on low heat for 30 minutes, or until the vegetables are tender.

Sprinkle the remaining ¼ cup Parmesan over the sauce before serving.

Makes 6 servings

Per serving: 135 calories, 3 g fat (20 % of calories), 6 g protein, 21 g carbohydrates, 6 g dietary fat, 5 mg cholesterol

Couscous with Tomato, Fennel, and Shrimp

1½ tablespoons olive oil

1 small onion, sliced

1 small bulb fennel, sliced

1 large clove garlic, minced

¼ teaspoon turmeric

2 cups water

⅓ pound cleaned raw salad shrimp

1 small tomato, peeled and chopped

2 tablespoons chopped fennel leaves

⅛ teaspoon ground black pepper

1½ cups couscous

In a large saucepan over medium heat, warm the oil. Add the onions, sliced fennel, and garlic and sauté for 5 minutes, or until the onions are soft. Stir in the turmeric and sauté for 1 minute.

Add the water to the pan and bring to a boil. Add the shrimp, return to a boil, and cook for 1 minute. Stir in the tomatoes, fennel leaves, pepper, and couscous. Remove from the heat. Cover and let stand for 5 minutes. Fluff with a fork before serving.

Makes 4 servings

Per serving: 354 calories, 6 g fat (16% of calories), 15.8 g protein, 57.7 g carbohydrates, 11.4 g dietary fiber, 58 mg cholesterol, 82 mg sodium

Chicken Risotto

Rice

¾ cup Arborio rice

2 teaspoons nondiet tub-style margarine or butter

2⅔ cups fat-free, reduced-sodium chicken broth

½ teaspoon dried thyme

½ teaspoon dried basil

¼ teaspoon ground black pepper

Chicken and Sauce

1 pound boneless, skinless chicken breast halves, cut into bite-size pieces

2 teaspoons nondiet tub-style margarine or butter

1 medium onion, chopped

⅓ cup fat-free, reduced-sodium chicken broth

1 clove garlic, minced

¼ teaspoon crushed saffron threads

1½ cups chopped broccoli florets and tender stems

½ red bell pepper, chopped

2 tablespoons grated Parmesan cheese

To make the rice: In a 2½-quart microwaveable baking dish, combine the rice and margarine or butter. Microwave on high power for 1 minute. Stir well.

Stir in the broth, thyme, basil, and black pepper. Cover and microwave for a total of 8 minutes; stop and stir after 4 minutes. Stir again after the full 8 minutes.

Microwave, uncovered, for 11 to 13 minutes, or until the rice is tender and most of the liquid is absorbed. Let stand for 3 minutes.

To make the chicken and sauce: While the rice is cooking, coat a large nonstick skillet with cooking spray. Place over medium heat and add the chicken. Cook, stirring occasionally, for 3 minutes, or until the chicken is tender. Remove from the pan.

In the same skillet, melt the margarine or butter. Add the onions, broth, garlic, and saffron and cook, stirring, for 5 minutes, or until the onions are tender.

Stir in the chicken, broccoli, and red peppers. Bring to a boil. Reduce the heat to medium-low, cover, and simmer, stirring frequently, for 6 to 7 minutes, or until the broccoli is crisp-tender.

Stir the chicken mixture into the rice. Sprinkle with the Parmesan.

Makes 4 servings

Per serving: 364 calories, 8.7 g total fat (22% of calories), 32.6 g protein, 37.4 g carbohydrates, 2.3 g dietary fiber, 71 mg cholesterol, 228 mg sodium

Curried Brown Rice with Mushrooms and Peas

   2 teaspoons peanut oil

   ½ cup chopped leeks (white part only)

   1½ teaspoons curry powder

   ½ cup sliced mushrooms

   1½ cups brown rice

   4 cups reduced-sodium vegetable broth

   1 cup frozen peas

   ½ cup chopped fresh cilantro

   1½ tablespoons reduced-sodium soy sauce

   ¼ teaspoon hot-pepper sauce

Preheat the oven to 350°.

In a large ovenproof saucepan over medium heat, warm the oil. Add the leeks and curry powder and sauté for 1 minute. Add the mushrooms and sauté for 3 minutes, or just until the leeks are soft and the mushrooms begin to release their liquid. Stir in the rice and cook for 1 minute.

Stir in the broth, peas, cilantro, soy sauce, and hot-pepper sauce and bring to a boil.

Cover the pan and bake for 40 to 50 minutes, or until the rice is tender and the liquid is absorbed. Let stand for 10 minutes. Fluff with a fork before serving.

Makes 4 servings

Per serving: 362 calories, 4.6 g fat (11% of calories), 9.7 g protein, 70.6 g carbohydrates, 6.2 g dietary fiber, 0 mg cholesterol, 327 mg sodium

Italian Wild Rice Pilaf

    2 teaspoons olive oil

    ½ cup wild rice, rinsed and drained

    ½ cup white rice

    2 cups fat-free, reduced-sodium chicken broth or water

    2 tablespoons pine nuts

    2 tablespoons chopped fresh basil

In a medium saucepan over medium heat, warm the oil. Add the wild rice and white rice and sauté for 30 seconds. Add the broth or water and bring to a boil. Cover, reduce the heat to low, and simmer for 20 minutes, or until most of the liquid is absorbed.

Meanwhile, preheat the oven to 400°. Coat a 1½-quart nonstick baking dish with cooking spray. Spoon the rice mixture into the prepared baking dish. Add the pine nuts and basil and stir well.

Bake for 10 to 15 minutes, or until the rice is tender and the liquid is absorbed.

Makes 4 servings

Per serving: 213 calories, 5.5 g fat (23% of calories), 7 g protein, 35 g carbohydrates, 0.5 g dietary fiber, 0 mg cholesterol, 35 mg sodium

Paella

 2 tablespoons olive oil

 3 cloves garlic, minced

 3 cups fat-free, reduced-sodium chicken broth

 1 can (14½ ounces) peeled whole tomatoes (with juice)

 ¼ teaspoon ground saffron or 8 saffron threads

 3 cups quick-cooking brown rice

 5 scallions, sliced

 1 small red bell pepper, sliced

12 peeled baby carrots

 ½ cup frozen peas, thawed

 ½ cup cooked or canned chickpeas

 4 water-packed artichoke hearts, halved

 ½ pound chicken tenders

 ⅓ pound low-fat smoked turkey sausage, sliced ½" thick

 8 littleneck clams, scrubbed

 8 mussels, scrubbed and beards removed

 ½ pound large shrimp (15 to 20 shrimp), peeled and deveined

Preheat the oven to 425°.

In a medium saucepan over medium-high heat, warm the oil. Add the garlic and sauté for 1 minute. Add the broth, tomatoes, and saffron and bring to a boil.

Meanwhile, spread the rice evenly over the bottom of a 10" × 13" non-stick baking dish. Add the scallions, peppers, carrots, peas, and chick-peas. Carefully pour the broth and tomatoes over the rice and vegetables and gently stir to coat. Top with the artichokes, chicken, and sausage.

Cover with foil and bake on the top rack of the oven for 10 minutes. Remove the foil and place the clams and mussels hinge side down in the rice. Top with the shrimp. Cover with the foil and return the dish to the top rack of the oven. Bake, covered, for 15 minutes, or until the clams and mussels open.

Remove and discard the foil. Bake, uncovered, for 5 minutes. Remove from the oven and let stand for 5 minutes before serving.

Makes 8 servings

Per serving: 458 calories, 9.6 g fat (19% of calories), 26.5 g protein, 65.9 g carbohydrates, 6.5 g dietary fiber, 85 mg cholesterol, 440 mg sodium

Pork Fried Rice

1 tablespoon peanut oil

4 scallions, thinly sliced

⅓ cup finely chopped celery

⅓ cup finely chopped red bell peppers

1 large clove garlic, minced

1 teaspoon minced fresh ginger

1 cup frozen peas

4 cups cooked rice

1 cup cubed fully cooked smoked ham

3 tablespoons reduced-sodium soy sauce

⅛ teaspoon ground black pepper

½ cup liquid egg substitute

Warm a wok or large nonstick skillet over medium-high heat. Add the oil and heat for 30 seconds, or until hot. Add the scallions, celery, and red peppers. Cook and stir for 4 minutes, or until the vegetables are tender.

Stir in the garlic, ginger, peas, rice, ham, soy sauce, and black pepper. Cook and stir for 5 minutes, or until heated through.

Pull the mixture to the sides of the wok and pour the egg substitute into the center. Cook, without stirring, for 2 to 3 minutes, or until set. Scrape the egg from the bottom of the wok and break it up. Stir it into the rice mixture until evenly combined.

Makes 4 servings

Per serving: 328 calories, 4.9 g fat (13% of calories), 16.5 g protein, 54.9 g carbohydrates, 2.2 g dietary fiber, 16 mg cholesterol, 792 mg sodium

Rice and Beans

2 cloves garlic, finely chopped

1 small onion, finely chopped

2 tablespoons olive oil

3 ribs celery, chopped

1 small green bell pepper, chopped

1 small red bell pepper, chopped

½ small green chile pepper, chopped

1 can (8 ounces) kidney beans, rinsed and drained

1 can (8 ounces) black beans, rinsed and drained

¼ cup fresh cilantro, chopped

Salt and freshly ground black pepper

3 cups hot cooked brown rice

Fat-free sour cream

Shredded low-fat sharp Cheddar cheese

In a large skillet over medium heat, sauté the garlic and onions in the oil.

Add the celery, green peppers, red peppers, and chile pepper and cook until soft.

Add the kidney beans, black beans, cilantro, salt, and pepper, and cook for 15 minutes.

Serve over the rice, garnished with the sour cream and Cheddar.

Makes 4 servings

Per serving: 219 calories, 7 g fat (29% of calories), 9 g protein, 30 g carbohydrates, 11 g dietary fiber, 0 mg cholesterol

Spanish Rice

1 tablespoon olive oil

⅛ teaspoon red-pepper flakes

¼ teaspoon ground cumin

1 cup chopped red or green bell peppers

1 cup sliced scallions

1 large clove garlic, minced

1 cup rice

¼ teaspoon dried oregano

2 cups fat-free, reduced-sodium chicken broth or vegetable broth, heated

2 cups Mexican-style stewed tomatoes (with juice)

1 tablespoon chopped fresh cilantro (optional)

In a large saucepan over medium heat, warm the oil. Add the red-pepper flakes and cumin and sauté for 2 minutes. Add the peppers, scallions, and garlic and sauté for 3 minutes, or just until the vegetables are tender.

Stir in the rice, oregano, and hot broth. Reduce the heat to low, cover, and simmer for 10 minutes, or until the broth is partially absorbed. Add the tomatoes (with juice). Cover and simmer, stirring occasionally, for 15 minutes, or until the rice is tender and the liquid is absorbed. Garnish with the cilantro (if using).

Makes 4 servings

Per serving: 276 calories, 4.3 g fat (14% of calories), 6.7 g protein, 52.7 g carbohydrates, 3 g dietary fiber, 0 mg cholesterol, 256 mg sodium

Wild Rice and Mushroom Pilaf

  1½ cups water

  ¾ cup wild rice, rinsed and drained

  1⅔ cups fat-free chicken broth

  1½ teaspoons olive oil

  2 small leeks (white part only), chopped

  ¾ cup sliced mushrooms

  1 teaspoon chopped fresh thyme

  ⅛ teaspoon ground black pepper

In a large saucepan over high heat, combine the water and rice. Bring to a boil. Cover, remove from the heat, and let stand for 20 minutes. Drain well and return to the pan.

Add 1½ cups of the broth and bring to a boil over medium-high heat. Reduce the heat to low, cover, and simmer for 25 minutes, or until the rice is tender and the liquid is absorbed.

Meanwhile, in a large nonstick skillet over medium heat, warm the oil. Add the leeks and sauté for 3 minutes. Add the mushrooms and thyme and sauté for 3 minutes. Add the pepper and the remaining broth. Cover and simmer for 5 minutes; set aside until the rice is ready.

Add the rice to the pan and mix well.

Makes 4 servings

Per serving: 154 calories, 2.2 g fat (13% of calories), 7.1 g protein, 28.1 g carbohydrates, 1.2 g dietary fiber, 0 mg cholesterol, 149 mg sodium

Baked Beans

    1 cup dried navy beans, soaked overnight

    2 cups water

    ⅓ cup crumbled low-fat turkey sausage

    ½ cup finely chopped onions

    1 cup fat-free, reduced-sodium chicken broth

    ¼ cup molasses

    2 tablespoons reduced-sodium ketchup

1½ teaspoons honey

1½ teaspoons brown sugar

1½ teaspoons brown mustard

1½ teaspoons Dijon mustard

    ½ teaspoon dry mustard

    ¼ teaspoon ground ginger

    ¼ teaspoon ground allspice

    Pinch of ground cloves

Drain the beans and place them in a large saucepan. Add the water and bring to a boil. Reduce the heat to medium-low and simmer for 1 hour, or until the beans are tender. Drain the beans and transfer to a 2-quart nonstick baking dish.

Meanwhile, in a medium saucepan over medium heat, cook and break up the sausage for 2 to 3 minutes, or until almost cooked through. Add the onions and sauté for 3 to 4 minutes, or until translucent. Stir the sausage mixture into the beans.

In the same pan over medium heat, combine the broth, molasses, ketchup, honey, brown sugar, brown mustard, Dijon mustard, dry mustard, ginger, allspice, and cloves. Bring to a simmer, stirring occasionally. Pour over the beans and mix well.

Preheat the oven to 300°. Cover and bake, stirring occasionally, for 1½ hours. Uncover and bake, stirring occasionally, for 45 minutes, or until the beans are tender and the sauce thickens.

Makes 4 servings

Per serving: 274 calories, 1.9 g fat (6% of calories), 14.5 g protein, 51.7 g carbohydrates, 0.6 g dietary fiber, 6 mg cholesterol, 176 mg sodium

NOTES:

- You may use other beans, such as baby lima, Great Northern, pinto, or pea beans, or a combination.

- This recipe can be doubled to serve 8. Use a 3-quart nonstick baking dish and increase the initial baking time to 2 hours.

VARIATIONS:

- *Baked Beans with Peppers:* Sauté 1 cup finely chopped red or green bell peppers along with the onions.

- *Vegetarian Baked Beans:* Replace the turkey sausage with tofu-based sausage. Or omit the sausage and sauté the onions in 2 teaspoons canola oil. Replace the chicken broth with vegetable broth.

Chickpea, Eggplant, and Tomato Casserole

1 eggplant, peeled and cubed

¼ cup fat-free, reduced-sodium chicken broth

1 medium onion, finely chopped

6 tomatoes, peeled, seeded, and chopped

¼ cup chopped fresh parsley

½ teaspoon dried thyme

1 bay leaf

2 cans (16 ounces each) chickpeas, rinsed
and drained

½ cup chopped fresh basil

2 teaspoons extra-virgin olive oil

½ teaspoon ground allspice

½ teaspoon red-pepper flakes

⅛ teaspoon ground black pepper

¼ cup grated reduced-fat Parmesan cheese

Lightly salt the eggplant and place in a colander for 15 minutes. Rinse and pat dry.

Preheat the oven to 400°. Coat a nonstick baking sheet with cooking spray. Place the eggplant on the baking sheet and bake for 20 minutes, turning occasionally. Remove from the oven and set aside.

Reduce the oven temperature to 375°.

In a large nonstick skillet over medium heat, warm the broth. Add the onions and cook, stirring occasionally, for 5 minutes. Stir in the tomatoes, parsley, thyme, and bay leaf. Cook and stir over medium-high heat until the liquid has evaporated. Remove from the heat. Remove and discard the bay leaf.

Stir in the eggplant, chickpeas, basil, oil, allspice, red-pepper flakes, and black pepper.

Coat a large nonstick baking dish with cooking spray. Spoon the eggplant mixture into the baking dish and sprinkle with the Parmesan. Bake for 30 minutes, or until bubbly and brown.

Makes 4 servings

Per serving: 466 calories, 5.7 g fat (11% of calories), 14.2 g protein, 93.2 g carbohydrates, 8 g dietary fiber, 0 mg cholesterol, 600 mg sodium

Chili con Carne

12 ounces extra-lean ground beef

2 cups chopped onions

1 cup chopped green peppers

3 cloves garlic, minced

1½ tablespoons chili powder

1 teaspoon ground cumin

1 teaspoon dried oregano

3 cans (8 ounces each) reduced-sodium tomato sauce

1 can (15 ounces) red kidney beans, rinsed and drained

1 can (14 ounces) whole tomatoes (with juice), coarsely chopped

1 tablespoon light brown sugar

Salt and ground black pepper

6 tablespoons shredded fat-free Cheddar cheese

2 scallions, thinly sliced

In a large saucepan over medium heat, brown the beef. Drain well, discarding the excess fat. Crumble the beef and set aside.

Return the pan to medium heat. Add the onions, peppers, and garlic and sauté for 5 minutes, or until the peppers are almost tender. Add the chili powder, cumin, and oregano and sauté for 2 to 3 minutes.

Add the beef, tomato sauce, beans, and tomatoes (with juice) and bring to a boil. Reduce the heat to medium-low, cover, and simmer for 10 minutes. Uncover and simmer until the desired consistency is reached.

Stir in the brown sugar and add the salt and pepper to taste.

Divide the chili among 6 serving bowls. Sprinkle each with the Cheddar and scallions.

Makes 6 servings

Per serving: 290 calories, 8.1 g fat (25% of calories), 22.6 g protein, 36.9 g carbohydrates, 8.9 g dietary fiber, 35 mg cholesterol, 376 mg sodium

NOTE:

• Always cook beef separately so the fat can be drained off.

VARIATIONS:

• *Chili Mole:* Sauté 1 small seeded and chopped jalapeño chile pepper (wear plastic gloves when handling) along with the green peppers. Replace the kidney beans with pinto or black beans. Stir in 2 to 3 tablespoons unsweetened cocoa powder along with the brown sugar. Omit the Cheddar cheese and scallions; garnish each serving with a dollop of fat-free sour cream and a sprinkling of finely chopped cilantro.

• *Eggplant Chili:* Sauté 1 cup peeled, cubed eggplant and 1 cup sliced carrots along with the green peppers. Replace the beef with 1½ cups cooked bulgur, barley, millet, rice, or crumbled firm tofu. Add to the mixture along with the tomatoes.

• *Mediterranean Chili con Carne:* Replace the beef with lean ground lamb. Replace the kidney beans with chickpeas. Omit the Cheddar cheese and scallions; garnish each serving with crumbled feta cheese and a sprinkling of sliced ripe olives.

Lima Bean Gratin

1 teaspoon olive oil

2 large shallots, chopped

¾ teaspoon dried thyme

1 can (15 ounces) lima beans, rinsed and drained

½ cup buttermilk

4 ounces feta cheese, crumbled

⅛ teaspoon ground nutmeg

2 tablespoons seasoned dry bread crumbs

1 tablespoon shredded Monterey Jack cheese

½ teaspoon paprika

In a medium nonstick skillet over medium heat, warm the oil. Add the shallots and thyme and sauté for 1 minute. Stir in the beans and sauté for 2 minutes.

Preheat the oven to 350°. Coat a gratin dish or shallow 1-quart nonstick baking dish with cooking spray and set aside.

Transfer half of the bean mixture to a food processor or blender and add the buttermilk, feta, and nutmeg. Process until smooth. Spoon the whole beans and pureed beans into the prepared baking dish and mix well.

In a small bowl, combine the bread crumbs, Monterey Jack, and paprika. Sprinkle over the casserole and bake for 8 to 10 minutes, or until golden.

Makes 4 servings

Per serving: 206 calories, 8.1 g fat (35% of calories), 11.6 g protein, 22.3 g carbohydrates, 0 g dietary fiber, 27 mg cholesterol, 712 mg sodium

Mexican Lentils with Peppers

2 teaspoons olive oil

¼ cup chopped scallions

¾ cup finely chopped carrots

1 cup finely chopped red bell peppers

1 cup finely chopped green bell peppers

½ cup rice

½ cup brown lentils, sorted and rinsed

½ teaspoon chili powder

½ teaspoon ground cumin

½ cup chopped tomatoes

2 cups fat-free chicken broth

In a medium saucepan over medium heat, warm the oil. Add the scallions, carrots, red peppers, and green peppers and sauté for 5 minutes, or until the vegetables are tender. Add the rice, lentils, chili powder and cumin and sauté for 2 minutes.

Stir in the tomatoes and broth and bring to a boil. Stir once and reduce the heat to low. Cover and simmer, stirring occasionally, for 25 minutes, or until the rice is tender and the liquid is absorbed.

Makes 4 servings

Per serving: 240 calories, 3.2 g fat (12% of calories), 11.5 g protein, 43.5 g carbohydrates, 3.4 g dietary fiber, 0 mg cholesterol, 185 mg sodium

NOTE:
- You can replace the green peppers with frozen peas. Add them halfway through the simmering time.

Savory Split Peas

2½ cups water

   1 cup green or yellow split peas, rinsed and drained

   6 medium red potatoes

   1 tablespoon olive oil

   1 cup finely chopped onions

   1 cup finely chopped red bell peppers

   1 teaspoon dried thyme

   ½ teaspoon dried rosemary, crumbled

   ¼ teaspoon ground black pepper

   ½ cup fat-free, reduced-sodium chicken broth

In a medium saucepan over medium-high heat, bring the water and split peas to a boil. Reduce the heat to low, cover, and simmer for 15 to 20 minutes, or until tender. Drain.

Meanwhile, place the potatoes in another medium saucepan with enough cold water to cover. Bring to a boil over medium-high heat and boil for 10 minutes. Drain. Cube the potatoes and set aside.

In a large saucepan over medium heat, warm the oil. Add the onions, red peppers, thyme, rosemary, and black pepper. Cook for 5 minutes, or until tender.

Add the potatoes and cook, stirring frequently, for 8 to 10 minutes, or until the potatoes are tender. Stir in the broth and split peas and cook for 5 to 7 minutes.

Makes 4 servings

Per serving: 324 calories, 4.4 g fat (12% of calories), 15.5 g protein, 58.5 g carbohydrates, 5.1 g dietary fiber, 0 mg cholesterol, 22 mg sodium.

Southwestern Black Beans

> 2 teaspoons canola oil
>
> 1 small red onion, chopped
>
> 1 clove garlic, minced
>
> 2 teaspoons chili powder
>
> 1 teaspoon ground cumin
>
> 2 cans (15 ounces each) black beans, rinsed and drained
>
> ¼ cup water or vegetable broth
>
> ¼ cup chopped fresh cilantro
>
> 2 tablespoons lime juice

In a large nonstick skillet over medium heat, warm the oil. Add the onions and sauté for 4 minutes, or until soft. Add the garlic, chili powder, and cumin and sauté for 1 minute.

Stir in the beans and water or broth. Cook, stirring occasionally, for 5 minutes, or until the beans are heated through and most of the liquid has evaporated.

Remove from the heat and stir in the cilantro and lime juice.

Makes 4 servings

Per serving: 209 calories, 4.6 g fat (20% of calories), 17.7 g protein, 39.7 carbohydrates, 13.1 g dietary fiber, 0 mg cholesterol, 680 mg sodium

All-American Meat Loaf

    2 cups shredded cabbage

    1 cup chopped onions

    1 cup shredded carrots

    ½ cup chopped green bell peppers

    2 cloves garlic, minced

    1 cup cooked brown rice or barley

    1 teaspoon dried basil

    ½ teaspoon dried savory

    ¼ teaspoon dried thyme

    1 pound extra-lean ground beef

    3 egg whites, lightly beaten

    ¾ teaspoon salt

    ¼ teaspoon ground black pepper

    Horseradish mustard

Preheat the oven to 350°. Coat an 8½" × 4½" × 2½" nonstick loaf pan with cooking spray.

Coat a large nonstick skillet with cooking spray and warm over medium heat. Add the cabbage, onions, carrots, green peppers, and garlic. Cover and cook, stirring occasionally, for 8 to 10 minutes, or until the carrots are tender. Stir in the rice or barley, basil, savory, and thyme. Let stand for 5 to 10 minutes, or until cool.

Add the beef, egg whites, salt, and pepper. Mix with your hands to combine. Pack the mixture into the prepared loaf pan.

Bake for about 1 hour, or until the juices run clear. Remove from the oven and set aside to cool for 5 minutes. Turn out of the pan onto a platter and slice. Serve with the horseradish mustard.

Makes 6 servings

Per serving: 165 calories, 7.2 g fat (39% of calories), 13.5 g protein, 11.5 g carbohydrates, 1.8 g dietary fiber, 35 mg cholesterol, 261 mg sodium

VARIATIONS:

- *Chili Sauce Meat Loaf:* Add ¼ cup chili sauce to the meat mixture. Spread 2 to 3 tablespoons chili sauce over the top of the loaf.

- *Cheesy Meat Loaf:* Add ½ cup shredded fat-free Cheddar cheese to the meat mixture. Sprinkle ¼ cup shredded fat-free Cheddar cheese over the top of the loaf during the last 10 minutes of baking.

- *Tofu Meat Loaf:* Replace the rice or barley with 1 cup pressed and crumbled tofu.

- *Ham Loaf:* Replace 8 ounces of the ground beef with 8 ounces ground lean baked ham. Replace the basil and savory with ¾ teaspoon crushed caraway seeds.

- *Pork-and-Beef Loaf:* Replace 8 ounces of the ground beef with 8 ounces ground pork tenderloin.

Microwave Sloppy Joes

   12 ounces extra-lean ground beef

    1 cup finely chopped onions

    1 large green bell pepper, chopped

    1 clove garlic, minced

    1 carrot, grated or finely shredded

    1 can (8 ounces) reduced-sodium tomato sauce

   ⅓ cup reduced-sodium ketchup

    2 teaspoons packed brown sugar

    2 teaspoons lemon juice

    1 teaspoon dried thyme

   ¼ teaspoon ground black pepper

   ¼ teaspoon salt (optional)

     Pinch of ground cinnamon

    4 English muffins or hamburger buns, split and toasted

In a 2½-quart microwaveable baking dish, combine the beef, onions, bell peppers, and garlic. Cover and microwave on high power for a total of 7 to 8 minutes, or until the beef is no longer pink; stop and stir every 3 minutes to break up the beef.

Break up any remaining large pieces of beef. Drain the mixture in a strainer or colander, then transfer to a large plate lined with paper towels. Blot the top of the mixture with additional paper towels. Return the mixture to the baking dish.

Stir in the carrots, tomato sauce, ketchup, brown sugar, lemon juice, thyme, black pepper, cinnamon, and salt (if using).

Cover and microwave on high power for 3 minutes, then stir. Microwave for 4 to 5 minutes, or until hot.

Serve over the English muffins or hamburger buns.

Makes 4 servings

Per serving: 381 calories, 11.5 g fat (27% of calories), 22.6 g protein, 46.4 g carbohydrates, 2.7 g dietary fiber, 53 mg cholesterol, 339 mg sodium

> NOTE:
>
> - You can replace the ground beef with ground turkey breast, ground chicken breast, or ground pork tenderloin that has been trimmed of all visible fat before grinding.

Pepper Steak

   2 cups sliced mushrooms

   1 cup sliced red bell peppers

   1 cup sliced green bell peppers

   2 cups sliced onions

   4 cloves garlic, minced

   1 pound boneless beef eye of round or sirloin tip steak, trimmed
     of all visible fat and cut into ¼"-thick strips

   2 teaspoons all-purpose flour

1½ cups fat-free, reduced-sodium beef broth

   ½ cup water

   ½ teaspoon dried thyme

   ½ cup tomato sauce

   1 tablespoon cornstarch

   ¼ cup dry white wine or nonalcoholic white wine

   1 tablespoon reduced-sodium Worcestershire sauce

     Salt and ground black pepper

   3 cups hot cooked brown rice

     Chopped fresh parsley

Coat a Dutch oven with cooking spray and warm over medium heat. Add the mushrooms, red peppers, and green peppers and sauté for 3 to 5 minutes, or until the peppers are tender. Remove the vegetables from the pan and set aside.

Add the onions and garlic to the pan and sauté for 2 to 3 minutes, or until the onions are tender. Coat the beef lightly with the flour. Add to the pan and cook over medium heat, stirring constantly, for 3 to 5 minutes. Add the broth, water, and thyme and bring to a boil. Reduce the heat, cover, and simmer for 30 to 35 minutes, or until the beef is tender. Add the tomato sauce and the reserved vegetables and cook for 5 to 10 minutes, or until the mixture is heated through.

In a small bowl, dissolve the cornstarch in the wine. Bring the beef mixture to a boil. Add the cornstarch mixture and boil, stirring constantly, until the mixture thickens. Add the Worcestershire sauce. Season to taste with the salt and pepper. Serve over the rice and garnish with the parsley.

Makes 4 servings

Per serving: 456 calories, 9.1 g fat (18% of calories), 34.7 g protein, 56.7 g carbohydrates, 6.9 g dietary fiber, 56 mg cholesterol, 258 mg sodium

VARIATIONS:

- *Asian Pepper Steak:* Replace the green peppers with 1 cup snow peas, steamed until crisp-tender. Add the snow peas, ½ cup sliced water chestnuts, and 1 teaspoon minced fresh ginger to the beef mixture along with the reserved mushrooms and red peppers. Replace the Worcestershire sauce with reduced-sodium soy sauce or teriyaki sauce.

- *Italian Pepper Steak:* Replace the green peppers and mushrooms with 1 cup chopped tomatoes and 1 cup sliced zucchini. Add ¾ to 1 teaspoon dried Italian herb seasoning. Serve over cooked fettuccine instead of rice. Garnish with chopped fresh basil instead of parsley.

- *Sweet-and-Sour Pepper Steak:* Stir ¼ cup apricot all-fruit spread and 3 to 4 teaspoons cider vinegar into the mixture at the end of the cooking time. Serve over steamed couscous instead of rice. Garnish with chopped fresh cilantro instead of parsley.

Peppers Stuffed with Beef and Spanish Rice

6 large green bell peppers

12 ounces extra-lean ground beef

1 large onion, finely chopped

⅔ cup chopped red bell peppers

1 can (8 ounces) tomato sauce

⅓ cup reduced-sodium ketchup

1½ cups cooked rice

1 tablespoon reduced-sodium Worcestershire sauce

2½ teaspoons chili powder

1¼ teaspoons dried marjoram

1 teaspoon paprika

½ teaspoon dry mustard

½ teaspoon dried thyme

¼ teaspoon celery salt

Cut the tops off the peppers, about 1" down. Remove the seeds and ribs, being careful not to rip the peppers. If necessary, trim the bottoms so that the peppers stand upright.

Choose a round, microwaveable baking dish large enough to hold the peppers upright in a circle around the edge. Coat the dish with cooking spray. Arrange the peppers upright in the dish and loosely cover with wax paper. Microwave on high power for a total of 4 minutes; stop and rotate the dish a quarter-turn after 2 minutes.

Lightly coat a large nonstick skillet with cooking spray. Add the beef, onions, and red peppers. Cook over medium-high heat, breaking up the beef with a spoon, until the beef is no longer pink and the peppers are tender. Drain the mixture in a strainer or colander, then transfer to a large plate lined with paper towels. Blot the top of the mixture with additional paper towels, then return to the skillet.

In a small bowl, combine the tomato sauce and ketchup. Add all but ¼ cup to the beef mixture. Stir the rice, Worcestershire sauce, chili powder, marjoram, paprika, mustard, thyme, and celery salt into the beef mixture.

Spoon equal amounts of the rice mixture into the green peppers. Drizzle the reserved tomato mixture on top of each pepper. Loosely cover with wax paper.

Microwave on high power for 4 to 6 minutes, or until the green peppers are just tender when pierced with a fork. Let stand for 5 minutes before serving.

Makes 6 servings

Per serving: 234 calories, 7.6 g fat (29% of calories), 14.3 g protein, 28.3 g carbohydrates, 3.5 g dietary fiber, 35 mg cholesterol, 335 mg sodium

VARIATIONS:

- *Mixed-Grain Stuffed Peppers:* Replace the cooked rice with a combination of cooked barley, bulgur, and quinoa.
- *Orzo-Stuffed Peppers:* Replace the cooked rice with 1½ cups cooked orzo pasta.

Skillet Goulash

    12 ounces extra-lean ground beef

    1 large red onion, finely chopped

    2 ribs celery, sliced

    1 large clove garlic, minced

  1½ cups fat-free, reduced-sodium beef broth

   ⅓ cup dry red wine or nonalcoholic red wine

    1 can (15 ounces) reduced-sodium tomato sauce

    2 cups thinly sliced red cabbage

    2 large carrots, sliced

    2 teaspoons paprika

    1 teaspoon dried thyme

   ¼ teaspoon dry mustard

   ¼ teaspoon ground black pepper

    1 large bay leaf

   12 ounces thin egg (no-yolk) noodles

   ¾ cup fat-free sour cream

    2 tablespoons chopped fresh parsley

Coat a large nonstick skillet with cooking spray and warm over medium heat. Add the beef and cook over medium-high heat, breaking up the beef with a spoon, for 7 to 8 minutes, or until no longer pink. Remove to a plate lined with paper towels. Blot the top with additional paper towels and set aside.

Drain any fat from the skillet and warm the skillet over medium-high heat. Add the onions, celery, and garlic and cook for 6 to 8 minutes, or until the celery is tender.

Stir in the broth, wine, and tomato sauce and mix well. Add the cabbage, carrots, paprika, thyme, mustard, pepper, and bay leaf. Bring to a boil. Reduce the heat to medium-low, cover, and simmer for 30 minutes, or until the carrots are tender. Remove and discard the bay leaf.

In a large pot of boiling water, cook the noodles according to package directions. Drain.

Reduce the heat to the lowest possible setting. Stir in the sour cream and gently heat through; do not boil. Serve over the noodles. Sprinkle with the parsley.

Makes 6 servings

Per serving: 365 calories, 9.3 g fat (22% of calories), 22.3 g protein, 48.1 g carbohydrates, 4.2 g dietary fiber, 35 mg cholesterol, 128 mg sodium

VARIATION:

- *Skillet Pork Goulash:* Replace the ground beef with ground pork tenderloin that has been trimmed of all visible fat before grinding.

Orange-Braised Pork Tenderloins

    4 pieces pork tenderloin (4 ounces each),
        trimmed of all visible fat

    ½ cup thinly sliced red onions

    1 navel orange, peeled and sectioned

    ½ cup orange juice

    ½ cup fat-free chicken broth

    1 tablespoon red wine vinegar

      Pinch of dried sage, crumbled

      Pinch of dried thyme

      Pinch of salt

Coat a large nonstick skillet with cooking spray and warm over medium-high heat. Sear the pork for 2 to 3 minutes per side, or until browned. Remove from the skillet and set aside.

Add the onions to the skillet and sauté for 2 minutes, or until soft. Add the vinegar and toss to coat. Add the oranges, orange juice, broth, sage, thyme, and salt. Reduce the heat to medium-low.

Return the pork to the skillet. Cover and cook for 8 to 10 minutes, or until the pork is only slightly pink in the center (check by inserting the tip of a sharp knife into 1 tenderloin).

Uncover and cook for 1 minute, or until the liquid is slightly reduced. Serve the pork with the oranges and sauce spooned over it.

Makes 4 servings

Per serving: 180 calories, 4.1 g fat (21% of calories), 24.9 g protein, 10.1 g carbohydrates, 1.3 g dietary fiber, 65 mg cholesterol, 89 mg sodium

Pork Chops with Apple-Raisin Relish

    4 pork chops (3 ounces each), trimmed of all visible fat
    ½ cup chopped sweet onions
    ¼ cup apple cider
        Pinch of ground cinnamon
        Pinch of ground nutmeg
    2 large red or green cooking apples, finely chopped
    2 tablespoons golden raisins
    2 teaspoons cider vinegar
    1 teaspoon maple syrup
        Pinch of salt

Coat a nonstick skillet with cooking spray and warm over medium-high heat for 2 minutes. Sear the pork chops for about 2 minutes per side, or until browned. Reduce the heat to medium and cook until the chops have only a trace of pink in the center (check by inserting the tip of a sharp knife into 1 chop).

Meanwhile, in a small saucepan, combine the onions, cider, cinnamon, and nutmeg. Simmer over low heat for 10 minutes. Add the apples and raisins and simmer for 5 minutes. Remove from the heat and stir in the vinegar, maple syrup, and salt. Serve with the pork chops.

Makes 4 servings

Per serving: 226 calories, 8.3 g fat (33% of calories), 18.9 g protein, 19.7 g carbohydrates, 2 g dietary fiber, 40 mg cholesterol, 43 mg sodium

VARIATION:

* *Chicken Thighs with Onion-Cranberry Relish:* Replace the pork chops with 8 boneless, skinless chicken thighs. Replace the raisins with dried cranberries. Increase the maple syrup to 2 teaspoons.

Lamb with Lemon Rice and Mint Sauce

Lamb

>   2 teaspoons minced garlic
>
>   1 teaspoon dried rosemary, crumbled
>
>   4 boneless lamb leg center steaks or loin lamb chops (4 ounces each), trimmed of all visible fat
>
>   Salt and ground black pepper

Rice

>   1½ cups fat-free, reduced-sodium chicken broth
>
>   ¾ cup rice
>
>   2 teaspoons grated lemon peel
>
>   1 tablespoon finely chopped fresh mint
>
>   Salt and ground black pepper

Sauce

>   ¼ cup packed light brown sugar
>
>   ¼ cup mint jelly
>
>   2–3 teaspoons finely chopped fresh mint

To make the lamb: In a small bowl, mash the garlic with the rosemary to make a paste. Rub evenly over the lamb and set aside to marinate for 30 minutes.

Coat a large nonstick skillet with cooking spray and warm over medium heat. Add the lamb and cook for about 4 minutes per side for medium doneness. Remove the lamb and place on a plate lined with paper towels. Blot the top with additional paper towels. Season the lamb to taste with the salt and pepper and set aside.

To make the rice: While the lamb is marinating, in a medium saucepan, bring the broth to a boil. Stir in the rice and lemon peel. Reduce the heat to low, cover, and simmer for about 25 minutes, or until the rice is tender and the liquid is absorbed. Stir in the mint. Season to taste with the salt and pepper.

To make the sauce: While the rice is cooking, combine the brown sugar and jelly in a small saucepan. Cook over medium heat until melted. Remove from the heat and stir in the mint. Serve warm with the lamb and rice.

Makes 4 servings

Per serving: 397 calories, 6.2 g fat (14% of calories), 27.4 g protein, 56.4 g carbohydrates, 0.5 g dietary fiber, 74 mg cholesterol, 91 mg sodium

VARIATIONS:

- *Lamb with Jalapeño Mint Sauce:* To make the lamb, replace the rosemary with finely chopped fresh cilantro. Omit the mint sauce. Instead, in a small saucepan, melt ½ cup jalapeño chile pepper jelly. Remove from the heat and stir in 2 teaspoons finely chopped fresh mint and 2 teaspoons finely chopped fresh cilantro. Serve the jalapeño mint sauce warm or at room temperature with the lamb and lemon rice.

- *Lamb with Mint Chutney:* Omit the mint sauce. Instead, in a small saucepan, combine ½ cup finely chopped fresh mint leaves, ¼ cup chopped onions, 2 tablespoons chopped dried apples, 2 tablespoons raisins, 1 teaspoon Dijon mustard, ¼ cup cider vinegar, ¼ cup packed light brown sugar, and ⅛ teaspoon salt. Cook over medium heat for 5 to 8 minutes, or until the liquid is absorbed. Serve the chutney warm or at room temperature with the lamb and lemon rice.

- *Pork Tenderloin with Honey-Mint Sauce:* Replace the lamb with 1 pound boneless pork tenderloin. Rub with the garlic-rosemary paste and let stand for 30 minutes. Cut into scant ½"-thick slices. Coat a medium nonstick skillet with cooking spray and warm over medium heat. Cook the pork for 3 to 4 minutes per side, or until browned. To make the honey-mint sauce, replace the brown sugar with honey.

Chicken-and-Bean Enchilada Casserole

¾ cup finely shredded reduced-fat Cheddar cheese

¾ cup finely shredded fat-free Cheddar cheese

4 boneless, skinless chicken breast halves (1 pound), cut into bite-size pieces

2 teaspoons olive oil

1 large onion, chopped

3 tablespoons fat-free chicken broth

2 cloves garlic, minced

1 large green bell pepper, chopped

1 can (15 ounces) reduced-sodium tomato sauce

1 cup mild picante sauce

1½ teaspoons ground cumin

1 teaspoon chili powder

1 can (15 ounces) no-salt-added kidney beans, rinsed and drained

10 corn tortillas (6" diameter)

½ cup fat-free sour cream

1 large tomato, chopped

Preheat the oven to 350°.

In a medium bowl, toss together the reduced-fat Cheddar and fat-free Cheddar.

Lightly coat a large nonstick skillet with cooking spray. Place over medium heat and add the chicken. Cook, stirring, for 10 minutes, or until the chicken is no longer pink. Remove and set aside.

Add the oil to the skillet and warm over medium heat. Add the onions, broth, and garlic. Cook, stirring, for 5 minutes, or until the onions are tender.

Stir in the peppers, tomato sauce, picante sauce, cumin, and chili powder. Add the chicken and beans and bring to a boil. Reduce the heat and simmer for 5 minutes.

Spread half of the chicken mixture evenly in a 9" × 13" nonstick baking dish. Place the tortillas on top, overlapping them to cover the entire surface. Sprinkle with half of the cheese mixture. Top with the remaining chicken mixture.

Cover with foil and bake for 30 to 35 minutes, or until heated through. Sprinkle with the remaining cheese mixture. Bake, uncovered, for 5 minutes, or until the cheese is partially melted.

To serve, use a sharp knife to cut the mixture into 8 pieces. Use a wide spatula to transfer the pieces to dinner plates. Top each serving with the sour cream and tomatoes.

Makes 8 servings

Per serving: 295 calories, 5.8 g fat (17% of calories), 26 g protein, 36 g carbohydrates, 4.2 g dietary fiber, 40 mg cholesterol, 552 mg sodium

Chicken Paprikash with Broccoli

> 4 boneless, skinless chicken breast halves (1 pound), cut into bite-size pieces
>
> ½ teaspoon salt (optional)
>
> ¼ teaspoon ground black pepper
>
> 1 large onion, chopped
>
> 1 clove garlic, minced
>
> ¾ cup fat-free chicken broth
>
> 2 teaspoons paprika
>
> 1 large red bell pepper, chopped
>
> 1½ cups broccoli florets
>
> 12 ounces egg (no-yolk) noodles
>
> 1 cup fat-free sour cream

Sprinkle the chicken with the salt (if using) and the black pepper.

Lightly coat a large nonstick skillet with cooking spray. Place over medium heat and add the chicken. Cook, stirring, for 7 to 8 minutes, or until the pieces begin to brown. Remove and set aside.

Add the onions, garlic, and 3 tablespoons of the broth to the skillet. Cook, stirring, for 5 minutes, or until the onions are tender. (If necessary, add more broth to prevent sticking.)

Stir in the paprika and cook for 1 minute. Stir in the remaining broth, then add the chicken, red peppers, and broccoli. Bring to a boil. Reduce the heat, cover, and simmer for 20 minutes, or until the vegetables are tender.

Meanwhile, cook the noodles according to the package directions. Drain, rinse with hot water, and drain again. If necessary, cover the noodles to keep warm.

Stir the sour cream into the chicken mixture. Cook, stirring, over low heat for 1 to 2 minutes, or until heated through. (Do not boil.) Serve the chicken over the noodles.

Makes 4 servings

Per serving: 470 calories, 6.5 g fat (12% of calories), 41.7 g protein, 64.1 g carbohydrates, 4.9 g dietary fiber, 69 mg cholesterol, 187 mg sodium

NOTE:

- For an interesting twist, replace the broccoli with broccoflower, a chartreuse-colored cross between broccoli and cauliflower. It is available in most supermarkets.

Chicken Piccata with Rice

    2 teaspoons olive oil

    4 boneless, skinless chicken breast halves (1 pound)

1½ cups quick-cooking brown rice

1¼ cups fat-free chicken broth

    ½ teaspoon dried oregano

    ¼ cup chopped fresh parsley

    ¼ cup lemon juice

    2 tablespoons capers, rinsed and chopped

    2 tablespoons chopped toasted pine nuts or almonds (see note)

Coat a large nonstick skillet with olive oil cooking spray. Add the oil and warm over medium heat. Add the chicken and cook for 5 minutes, or until lightly browned on both sides. Add the rice, broth, oregano, parsley, lemon juice, and capers. Bring to a boil. Cover and simmer over medium-low heat for 10 minutes, or until the chicken is cooked through. Remove from the heat and let stand for 5 minutes. Sprinkle with the pine nuts or almonds.

Makes 4 servings

Per serving: 449 calories, 9.8 g fat (20% of calories), 33.6 g protein, 56.3 g carbohydrates, 4.1 g dietary fiber, 69 mg cholesterol, 329 mg sodium

NOTE:

    • To toast the nuts, place them in a dry nonstick skillet over medium heat. Toast the nuts, shaking the skillet often, for 3 to 5 minutes, or until fragrant and golden.

New American Fried Chicken

½ cup buttermilk

½ cup fresh white bread crumbs

½ cup fresh whole wheat bread crumbs

½ teaspoon paprika

1 teaspoon ground black pepper

½ teaspoon dried thyme or sage

1 tablespoon chopped fresh parsley

  Pinch of salt (optional)

4 whole chicken legs

Coat a rack with cooking spray. Place the rack on a foil-lined baking sheet and set aside. Preheat the oven to 425°.

Place the buttermilk in a shallow dish. Place the bread crumbs in another shallow dish. In a cup or small bowl, combine the paprika, pepper, thyme or sage, parsley, and salt (if using). Add 1 teaspoon to the bread crumbs and the remainder to the buttermilk.

Dip the chicken pieces in the buttermilk to coat, then roll them in the seasoned bread crumbs to coat. Place the chicken on the prepared rack and lightly coat with cooking spray.

Bake for 15 minutes. Turn the chicken and coat again with cooking spray. Bake for 15 minutes, or until the crust is golden brown and the juices run clear when the joint is pierced.

Makes 4 servings

Per serving: 226 calories, 8.8 g fat (36% of calories), 27.9 g protein, 7.5 g carbohydrates, 0.3 g dietary fiber, 90 mg cholesterol, 178 mg sodium

Roast Chicken with Winter Vegetables

1 broiler-fryer chicken (about 3 pounds)

1 clove garlic, minced

2 teaspoons crushed fennel seeds

4 small red potatoes, quartered

3 medium carrots, halved and quartered

2 small turnips, peeled and quartered

1 small onion, quartered

¼ teaspoon salt

½ cup fat-free, reduced-sodium chicken broth or water

Preheat the oven to 400°. Coat a rack and a shallow roasting pan with olive oil cooking spray and set aside.

Rinse the chicken and pat dry with paper towels. Remove and discard any excess fat from inside the chicken. Starting at the neck opening, use your fingers to gently loosen the skin from the meat and create a pocket on each side of the breast. Leave the skin attached to the breastbone.

Rub the garlic and ½ teaspoon of the fennel seeds onto the meat underneath the skin. Place the chicken, breast side up, on the prepared rack in the roasting pan.

In a shallow bowl, combine the potatoes, carrots, turnips, and onions. Coat lightly with olive oil cooking spray. Sprinkle with the remaining 1½ teaspoons fennel seeds and the salt and toss to coat. Loosely stuff some of the vegetables into the chicken cavity. Place the remaining vegetables in the pan around the chicken. Skewer the neck skin to the back of the chicken and tie the legs to the tail. Insert a meat thermometer in the thickest part of a thigh.

Roast for 30 minutes. Turn the vegetables and roast for about 30 minutes, or until the thermometer registers 180° to 185° and the chicken is no longer pink.

Transfer the vegetables from the pan to an ovenproof serving dish; keep warm in the oven on low heat. Let the chicken stand for 10 minutes before carving.

Meanwhile, pour all of the fat from the roasting pan and discard. Add the broth or water to the pan, scraping with a pancake turner to remove browned particles. Pour the pan juices into a small saucepan and cook at a brisk simmer for 3 to 4 minutes, or until reduced slightly.

Remove the skin from the chicken and discard. Serve the chicken and vegetables with the pan juices.

Makes 6 servings

Per serving: 247 calories, 4.5 g fat (16% of calories), 19.4 g protein, 32.9 g carbohydrates, 1.1 g dietary fiber, 49 mg cholesterol, 181 mg sodium

NOTE:

- The technique of seasoning poultry breast with garlic and herbs before roasting can also be applied to Cornish game hens or bone-in chicken breasts. Another aromatic option is to place lemon, lime, or orange slices under the skin.

Texas-Style Chicken Fajitas

1 clove garlic, minced

½ teaspoon ground cumin

½ teaspoon chili powder

¼ teaspoon reduced-sodium Worcestershire sauce

12 ounces boneless, skinless chicken breasts, cut into short strips

½ cup chopped fresh cilantro

3 medium red or green bell peppers, cut into short strips

1 medium red onion, thinly sliced and separated into rings

3 tablespoons lime juice

8 warm corn tortillas (6" diameter)

8 tablespoons fat-free sour cream

8 tablespoons salsa

In a medium bowl, stir together the garlic, cumin, chili powder, and Worcestershire. Stir in the chicken and cilantro until coated. Cover and refrigerate for 1 hour.

Coat a large nonstick skillet with cooking spray and warm over medium-high heat until hot. Add the chicken and cilantro and cook, stirring, for 3 to 4 minutes, or until the chicken is no longer pink. Transfer to a large bowl and keep warm.

Add the peppers to the skillet. Cook, stirring, for 4 to 6 minutes, or until the peppers are crisp-tender. Transfer to the bowl with the chicken.

Add the onions to the skillet. Cook, stirring, for about 3 minutes, or until the onions are crisp-tender.

Return the chicken and peppers to the skillet. Drizzle the lime juice over the mixture and stir until combined. Remove from the heat.

To serve, place the mixture on the tortillas. Garnish each tortilla with 1 tablespoon of the sour cream and 1 tablespoon of the salsa. Roll up to enclose the filling. Serve immediately.

Makes 4 servings

Per serving: 312 calories, 4.1 g fat (12% of calories), 27.2 g protein, 44.5 g carbohydrates, 4.3 g dietary fiber, 52 mg cholesterol, 377 mg sodium

NOTE:

- Fajitas come in many flavors. If you like, replace the chicken with lean flank steak, beef tenderloin, pork tenderloin, swordfish, halibut, or medium shrimp. The cooking time for fish and shrimp is comparable to that for chicken. The cooking time for meat will be 2 to 3 minutes longer.

Barbecued Turkey Sandwiches

   1 pound turkey breast cutlets, pounded ¼" thick and cut into short, thin strips

   ¼ teaspoon dried thyme

   ¼ teaspoon ground black pepper

   ¼ teaspoon salt (optional)

   2 teaspoons nondiet tub-style margarine or butter

   1 medium onion, chopped

   1 small green bell pepper, chopped

   1 small clove garlic, minced

   ½ cup reduced-sodium ketchup

   ¼ cup water

   1 tablespoon reduced-sodium Worcestershire sauce

   1 tablespoon honey

   ¼ teaspoon dry mustard

     Pinch of ground allspice

   4 Kaiser rolls

Season the turkey with the thyme, black pepper, and salt (if using).

In a large nonstick skillet over medium heat, melt the margarine or butter. Cook the turkey for 2 minutes per side, or until lightly browned. Remove and set aside.

Coat a large nonstick skillet with cooking spray and warm over medium heat. Add the onions, green peppers, and garlic and cook, stirring occasionally, for 5 to 6 minutes, or until the peppers are soft. If necessary, add 1 tablespoon of water to the skillet to prevent sticking.

Stir in the ketchup, water, Worcestershire sauce, honey, mustard, and allspice. Simmer for 10 minutes, or until the vegetables are tender.

Add the turkey, reduce the heat to very low, and cook for 5 minutes, or until the turkey is heated through and flavored with the sauce. Spoon onto rolls just before serving.

Makes 4 servings

Per serving: 378 calories, 5.2 g fat (13% of calories), 33.8 g protein, 48.5 g carbohydrates, 1.5 g dietary fiber, 75 mg cholesterol, 417 mg sodium

NOTE:

- For a Carolina-style accompaniment, top the turkey barbecue with coleslaw made with a reduced-fat oil-and-vinegar dressing.

Turkey-and-Bean Burritos

1 pound ground turkey breast

1 medium onion, chopped

1 clove garlic, minced

1 can (15 ounces) no-salt-added kidney beans, rinsed and
drained

1 can (8 ounces) reduced-sodium tomato sauce

⅓ cup picante sauce

1½ teaspoons chili powder

⅛ teaspoon salt (optional)

1 cup shredded fat-free Cheddar cheese

¾ cup shredded reduced-fat sharp Cheddar cheese

10 flour tortillas (8" diameter)

Preheat the oven to 375°.

Coat a large saucepan with cooking spray and warm over medium
heat. Add the turkey, onions, and garlic and sauté for 8 to 10 minutes,
or until the turkey is no longer pink. If necessary, add a small amount
of water to the pan to prevent sticking.

Stir in the beans, tomato sauce, picante sauce, chili powder, and salt (if
using). Cover and cook, stirring occasionally, over low heat for 10 minutes.

In a small bowl, toss together the fat-free Cheddar and reduced-fat
Cheddar.

Coat a nonstick baking sheet with cooking spray.

Place a tortilla on a flat work surface. Spoon a generous ½ cup of
the turkey mixture onto the tortilla, positioning it slightly off-cen-
ter. Sprinkle with a scant 2 tablespoons of the cheese mixture.
Carefully roll up the tortilla and place, seam side down, on the pre-

pared baking sheet. Repeat with the remaining tortillas, turkey mixture, and cheese.

Bake for 12 to 14 minutes, or until the cheese is mostly melted and the
tortillas begin to crisp around the edges.

Makes 10 servings

Per serving: 231 calories, 4.3 g fat (17% of calories), 20.9 g protein, 26.6 g carbohydrates, 1.4 g
dietary fiber, 34 mg cholesterol, 445 mg sodium

NOTES:

- If you have extra picante sauce, it makes a delicious topping for the
  burritos.
- This recipe makes enough for a generous supply of leftovers. To reheat for lunch, a snack, or a second dinner, place one burrito at a
  time on a microwaveable plate. Cover it with wax paper and microwave on high power for 30 to 40 seconds, or until heated through.

Turkey and Sausage Jambalaya

    2 teaspoons canola oil
    1 cup chopped scallions
    1 large rib celery, sliced
    1 small red or green bell pepper, coarsely chopped
    ⅓ cup chopped fresh parsley
    1 pound boneless, skinless turkey breast, cut into ¾" cubes
    2 cups fat-free chicken broth
 1¼ cups quick-cooking rice
    ½ cup chopped low-fat smoked turkey sausage
    ½ teaspoon dried thyme
    ¼ teaspoon ground red pepper
    ⅛ teaspoon ground black pepper
    1 large bay leaf
    1 can (16 ounces) chopped tomatoes (with juice)

In a large nonstick skillet over medium heat, warm the oil. Add the scallions, celery, red or green peppers, and parsley. Cook, stirring, for 3 minutes, or until the onions are tender.

Add the turkey and cook, stirring, for 4 minutes. Stir in the broth, rice, sausage, thyme, red pepper, black pepper, and bay leaf. Bring to a simmer. Reduce the heat and gently simmer, stirring occasionally, for 3 minutes.

Stir in the tomatoes (with juice) and cook just until the mixture comes to a simmer. Turn off the heat, cover, and let stand for 5 minutes.

Remove and discard the bay leaf. Stir well.

Makes 6 servings

Per serving: 231 calories, 3.3 g fat (13% of calories), 24.4 g protein, 25.1 g carbohydrates, 2.3 g dietary fiber, 56 mg cholesterol, 415 mg sodium

Blackened Catfish

1 cup quick-cooking white or brown rice

2 cups water

1 medium tomato, finely chopped

¼ cup minced scallions

¼ teaspoon salt

Pinch of dried thyme

4 catfish fillets (4 ounces each and ½" thick)

2 tablespoons Cajun seasoning

In a medium saucepan, combine the rice, water, tomatoes, scallions, salt, and thyme. Bring to a boil. Cover, reduce the heat to low, and cook for about 10 minutes, or until the rice is tender and the liquid is absorbed.

Meanwhile, heat a large cast-iron skillet on high heat for about 8 minutes, or until it is very hot (see note).

Coat the catfish with olive oil cooking spray. Rub in the Cajun seasoning, coating each piece well. Place the catfish in the skillet and cook for about 2 minutes per side, or until the fish is opaque and flakes easily when tested with a fork. Serve over the rice.

Makes 4 servings

Per serving: 236 calories, 7.5 g fat (29% of calories), 19.2 g protein, 21.6 g carbohydrates, 0.9 g dietary fiber, 58 mg cholesterol, 487 mg sodium

NOTE:

• The blackening process creates some smoke, so use an exhaust fan or cook the fish outdoors on a very hot grill. Be careful when handling the skillet after cooking because it takes considerable time to cool down.

VARIATION:

• *Oven-Blackened Catfish:* Bake the seasoned catfish at 400° for about 20 minutes, or until the fish is opaque and flakes easily when tested with a fork. Serve with hot cooked orzo pasta.

Orange Roughy Caribbean

   1 cup fish stock or fat-free chicken broth

   1 yellow bell pepper, cut into thin strips

   8 scallions, sliced diagonally into 1" pieces

   4 slices lime

   1 tablespoon chopped fresh cilantro

   ¼ teaspoon curry powder

   4 skinless orange roughy fillets (4 ounces each and ½" thick)

   4 cups hot cooked rice

In a large nonstick skillet, combine the stock or broth, peppers, scallions, lime slices, cilantro, and curry powder. Cover and bring to a boil.

Carefully add the orange roughy. Reduce the heat to medium-low, cover, and gently simmer for 5 to 6 minutes, or until the orange roughy is opaque and flakes easily when tested with a fork. Discard the lime slices.

Serve with the rice and top with the pepper and scallion sauce.

Makes 4 servings

Per serving: 305 calories, 1.4 g fat (4% of calories), 22.3 g protein, 49.2 g carbohydrates, 0.3 g dietary fiber, 22 mg cholesterol, 156 mg sodium

NOTES:

- You can replace the yellow pepper with red, orange, or green bell peppers, or a colorful combination.
- To cut the scallions diagonally, hold a sharp knife at a 45-degree angle to the scallion and make evenly spaced cuts.

Stuffed Flounder

½ bag (8 ounces) fresh spinach
½ shallot, finely chopped
1½ teaspoons olive oil
4 flounder fillets (4 ounces each)
Salt and freshly ground black pepper
4 ounces Monterey Jack cheese, grated

Preheat the oven to 350°. Lightly coat a baking dish with cooking spray and set aside.

In a medium saucepan over medium heat, blanch the spinach in boiling salted water for about 2 minutes. Let cool, drain, and squeeze out the excess water.

In a small skillet, sauté the shallots in the olive oil.

Place the flounder on a board and salt and pepper each side of the fillets. Layer an equal amount of spinach, shallots, and cheese on each fillet. Roll up the fillets and place the rolls, seam side down, in the prepared baking dish. Bake for about 15 to 20 minutes, or until the fish flakes easily when tested with a fork.

Makes 4 servings
Per roll: 270 calories, 10 g fat (33% of calories), 41 g protein, 5 g carbohydrates, 2 g dietary fiber, 107 mg cholesterol

Teriyaki Tuna

¼ cup reduced-sodium soy sauce

3 tablespoons dry sherry or nonalcoholic white wine

1 tablespoon sesame oil

2 teaspoons packed brown sugar

¾ teaspoon ground ginger

2–3 drops hot-pepper sauce

4 tuna steaks (4 ounces each, ½"–¾" thick)

In a shallow bowl, combine the soy sauce, sherry or wine, oil, brown sugar, ginger, and hot-pepper sauce. Add the tuna and turn to coat both sides. Cover with plastic wrap and marinate in the refrigerator, turning the pieces occasionally, for at least 1 hour.

Preheat the broiler. Coat the rack of a broiler pan with cooking spray. Remove the tuna from the marinade and place on the rack. Drizzle with a few tablespoons of the marinade.

Broil 4" from the heat for 3 minutes. Using a wide spatula, turn the tuna and drizzle with a few more tablespoons of the marinade. Discard the remaining marinade. Broil for 2 to 5 minutes, or until the tuna is opaque and flakes easily when tested with a fork.

Makes 4 servings

Per serving: 152 calories, 2.8 g fat (17% of calories), 26.5 g protein, 2.3 g carbohydrates, 0 g dietary fiber, 49 mg cholesterol, 306 mg sodium

NOTES:

• You can replace the tuna with swordfish or mahi mahi.

Crab Cakes

8 ounces lump or backfin crabmeat, flaked

1 cup soft white or whole wheat bread crumbs

1 tablespoon chopped onion

1 tablespoon chopped celery

1 tablespoon chopped red bell pepper

1 tablespoon chopped fresh parsley

1 egg, lightly beaten

1 egg white, lightly beaten

2 teaspoons reduced-sodium Worcestershire sauce

1 teaspoon lemon juice

⅛ teaspoon ground black pepper

½ teaspoon hot-pepper sauce

2 teaspoons canola oil

In a medium bowl, combine the crabmeat, bread crumbs, onions, celery, bell peppers, parsley, egg, egg white, Worcestershire sauce, lemon juice, black pepper, and hot-pepper sauce. Cover and refrigerate for 30 minutes to make handling easier.

Shape the crab mixture into 4 cakes.

In a large nonstick skillet over medium-high heat, warm the oil. Add the crab cakes and cook for 5 to 7 minutes per side, or until golden.

Makes 4 servings

Per serving: 87 calories, 4.1 g fat (43% of calories), 5.3 g protein, 6.9 g carbohydrates, 0.5 g dietary fiber, 62 mg cholesterol, 134 mg sodium

NOTE:

• Mustard mayonnaise makes an excellent topping for these crab cakes. Combine 2½ teaspoons Dijon mustard with ¼ cup fat-free mayonnaise.

Broiled Sea Scallops with Ginger

> 1 pound sea scallops
> 1 small piece fresh ginger, peeled
> 1 clove garlic, finely chopped
>   Juice of 1 lime
> ¼ cup chopped fresh parsley

Preheat the broiler.

Rinse the scallops and pat them dry. Arrange them in the broiler pan. Grate the ginger over the scallops, then sprinkle with the garlic and lime juice.

Broil for 8 minutes, or until the scallops turn white and opaque. (Do not overcook.) Sprinkle with the parsley before serving.

Makes 4 servings

109 calories, 1 g fat (1% of calories), 19 g protein, 6 g carbohydrates, 0 g dietary fiber, 37 mg cholesterol

NOTE:

- Serve with steamed asparagus, a green salad, and whole wheat couscous for optimal fiber Sparks.

Skinny Shrimp Scampi

1 cup quick-cooking brown rice

1 pound extra-large shrimp (26 to 30 shrimp), peeled and deveined, tails attached

1 tablespoon olive oil

8 slices lemon

8 scallions, trimmed and cut into ½" pieces

4 cloves garlic, minced

½ cup freshly squeezed orange juice

½ cup chopped fresh parsley

¼ teaspoon ground black pepper

Cook the rice according to the package directions. Set aside and keep warm.

Meanwhile, cut a 1" lengthwise slit in each shrimp, starting at the head; set aside.

In a large nonstick skillet over medium-high heat, warm the oil for 1 minute. Add the lemon slices and scallions and sauté for 3 minutes. Add the garlic and cook for 1 minute. Transfer the lemons, scallions, and garlic to a small bowl; set aside.

Add the shrimp to the skillet and cook for 2 to 3 minutes, or until they start to turn opaque. Add the orange juice, parsley, and pepper and bring to a boil. Return the lemons, scallions, and garlic to the skillet and cook for 2 minutes. Serve hot over the rice.

Makes 4 servings

Per serving: 318 calories, 5.9 g fat (17% of calories), 23.4 g protein, 43.3 g carbohydrates, 3.4 g dietary fiber, 175 mg cholesterol, 207 mg sodium

VARIATION:

• *Sea-Scallop Scampi:* Replace the shrimp with sea scallops.

Shrimp-and-Vegetable Stir-Fry

1 small head bok choy

¾ cup fish stock or fat-free chicken broth

1 tablespoon reduced-sodium soy sauce

1 teaspoon sesame oil

¾ pound large shrimp (23 to 30 shrimp), peeled, deveined, and tails removed

1 clove garlic, minced

1 cup baby carrots, halved lengthwise

4 scallions, trimmed and sliced diagonally into 1" pieces

1 red bell pepper, cut into strips

½ cup canned sliced water chestnuts, drained

8 ears canned baby corn

2 teaspoons cornstarch

3 cups hot cooked brown rice

Trim and discard the root end of the bok choy. Cut off and discard most of the green leaves. Cut into diagonal slices and set aside.

In a measuring cup, combine the stock or broth, soy sauce, and oil. Stir to blend thoroughly.

Heat a dry wok or large nonstick skillet over high heat for 5 minutes. Add 2 tablespoons of the broth mixture and heat for 1 minute. Add the shrimp and stir-fry briskly for 30 seconds. Cover and cook for 2 minutes, or until the shrimp start to turn opaque. Transfer the shrimp and pan juices to a bowl and set aside.

Return the wok or skillet to high heat for 1 minute. Add 2 tablespoons of the broth mixture. Add the garlic and cook for 30 seconds.

Add the bok choy, carrots, scallions, and peppers. Stir-fry for 3 minutes, or until the vegetables are just crisp-tender. Add the water chestnuts and corn and stir-fry for 30 seconds. Add the reserved shrimp and pan juices.

Combine the cornstarch with the remaining ½ cup of the broth mixture and mix well. Add to the wok or skillet and stir-fry to coat all of the ingredients. Cover and cook, stirring once, for 3 minutes, or until thick. Serve immediately with the rice.

Makes 4 servings

Per serving: 319 calories, 3.7 g fat (10% of calories), 22.6 g protein, 50 g carbohydrates, 5.5 g dietary fiber, 131 mg cholesterol, 469 mg sodium

VARIATION:

- *Scallop-and-Vegetable Stir-Fry:* Replace the shrimp with sea scallops.

Black-Bean Casserole with Cornbread Topping

Casserole

   1 tablespoon olive oil

   1 cup chopped onions

   1 large clove garlic, minced

   1 large green bell pepper, seeded and finely chopped

   1 large rib celery, finely chopped

   1 medium carrot, finely chopped

   1 can (15 ounces) black beans, rinsed and drained

   1 cup drained canned diced tomatoes with green chiles

   ½ teaspoon dried oregano

   ½ cup packed chopped fresh cilantro

Topping

   1 cup yellow cornmeal

   ⅓ cup unbleached white flour

   ½ teaspoon baking powder

   ¼ teaspoon baking soda

   ¼ teaspoon salt

   ½ cup fresh or frozen corn

   1 cup buttermilk

   1 tablespoon canola oil

   1 tablespoon maple syrup

To make the casserole: Preheat the oven to 400°. Coat a shallow oven-proof baking dish (approximately 8" round by 2" deep) with vegetable cooking spray. Set aside.

In a nonreactive nonstick skillet over medium heat, warm the oil. Add the onions and garlic. Sauté for 2 minutes. Add the peppers, celery, and carrots. Sauté for 5 minutes. Add the beans, tomatoes, and oregano. Cook for 5 minutes, or until the vegetables begin to soften. Remove from the heat, stir in the cilantro, and transfer to the prepared baking dish. Set aside.

To make the topping: In a large bowl, combine the cornmeal, flour, baking powder, baking soda, and salt. Stir in the corn.

In a separate bowl, whisk together the buttermilk, oil, and maple syrup. Add to the cornmeal mixture and stir just until blended. Pour over the bean mixture and bake for 30 to 35 minutes, or until a wooden pick inserted in the center of the cornbread comes out clean. Cut into wedges and serve.

Makes 4 servings

Per serving: 393 calories, 9.8 g fat (20% of calories), 16.4 g protein, 69.6 g carbohydrates, 13.7 g dietary fiber, 2 mg cholesterol, 678 mg sodium

NOTES:
- For a spicier dish, add ½ teaspoon seeded and chopped jalapeño chile peppers (wear plastic gloves when handling) along with the celery and carrots. Or add hot-pepper sauce to taste.
- If desired, puree half of the cooked bean mixture in a food processor or blender. Stir into the remaining bean mixture and mix well before transferring to the prepared baking dish.

Broccoli and Red Pepper Stir-Fry

½ cup reduced-sodium vegetable broth

1½ tablespoons black bean garlic sauce

1 tablespoon reduced-sodium soy sauce

1 tablespoon cornstarch

2 teaspoons rice-wine vinegar

1 teaspoon toasted sesame oil

¼ teaspoon red-pepper flakes

1 tablespoon peanut oil

3 cups broccoli florets

1 tablespoon water

1 medium red bell pepper, cut into small strips

2 cloves garlic, minced

1 teaspoon minced fresh ginger

4 cups hot cooked rice

In a small bowl, whisk together the broth, garlic sauce, soy sauce, cornstarch, vinegar, sesame oil, and red-pepper flakes. Set aside.

Warm a wok or large nonstick skillet over high heat. Add the peanut oil and tilt the pan in all directions to coat. Add the broccoli and stir-fry for 10 seconds. Add the water, cover, and steam, shaking the pan occasionally, for 30 to 45 seconds, or until the broccoli is just crisp-tender.

Add the red peppers, garlic, and ginger; stir-fry for 30 seconds, or until the peppers are just crisp-tender.

Quickly whisk the sauce and pour it into the pan. Cook and stir for 20 seconds, or just until thickened. Serve over the rice.

Makes 4 servings

Per serving: 304 calories, 5.6 g fat (16% of calories), 7.7 g protein, 56.6 g carbohydrates, 3.3 g dietary fiber, 0 mg cholesterol, 173 mg sodium

Chickpea Burgers

  1 can (16 ounces) chickpeas, rinsed, drained, and mashed

  ½ cup finely chopped red onions

  ½ cup finely chopped celery

  1 cup unseasoned dry bread crumbs

  ½ cup reduced-sodium tomato sauce

  1 tablespoon Dijon mustard

  1 tablespoon Worcestershire sauce

  1 egg white

  ½ teaspoon liquid smoke (optional)

  2 teaspoons olive oil

  1 teaspoon dried thyme

  ¼–¾ teaspoon salt

  ¼ teaspoon ground black pepper

  ½ cup chopped fresh parsley

Preheat the oven to 350°. In a large bowl, combine the chickpeas, onions, celery, bread crumbs, tomato sauce, mustard, Worcestershire sauce, egg white, liquid smoke (if using), olive oil, thyme, salt, pepper, and parsley. Mix well. Using your hands, shape the mixture into 4 patties.

Place the patties on a nonstick baking sheet. Cover with aluminum foil and bake for 30 minutes. Uncover and bake for 5 to 10 minutes, or until the patties are lightly browned.

Makes 4 servings

Per serving: 266 calories, 6 g fat (20% of calories), 10.6 g protein, 43.3 g carbohydrates, 6.3 g dietary fiber, 0 mg cholesterol, 789 mg sodium

Spinach-Cheese Enchiladas

> 2 cups reduced-sodium vegetable broth
>
> 1 cup chopped canned green chile peppers
>
> 2 tomatoes, peeled and finely chopped
>
> 2 tablespoons finely chopped scallions
>
> 2 cloves garlic, minced
>
> 2 tablespoons cornstarch
>
> 2 tablespoons water
>
> 1¼ pounds fresh spinach, coarsely chopped
>
> ½ cup shredded reduced-fat Monterey Jack cheese
>
> 8 corn tortillas (6" diameter)

Preheat the oven to 400°. Coat a 9" × 13" nonstick baking dish with cooking spray and set aside.

In a medium saucepan, combine the broth, peppers, tomatoes, scallions, and garlic. Bring to a boil over high heat. Reduce the heat to medium and simmer for 15 minutes.

In a glass measuring cup, whisk together the cornstarch and water. Add to the tomato mixture. Cook and stir until thickened. Remove from the heat.

While the sauce is cooking, place the spinach in a large saucepan with about 2 tablespoons water. Cover and steam over medium heat for 2 to 4 minutes, or until the spinach is wilted. Divide the spinach and Monterey Jack evenly among the tortillas. Roll up to enclose the filling.

Place the enchiladas seam side down in a single layer in the prepared baking dish. Top with the tomato mixture. Bake for 10 minutes, or until the filling is hot.

Makes 4 servings

Per serving: 240 calories, 4.5 g fat (16% of calories), 12.8 g protein, 41.3 g carbohydrates, 5.1 g dietary fiber, 10 mg cholesterol, 749 mg sodium

Spinach-and-Mushroom Frittata

½ cup chopped onions

4 ounces mushrooms, sliced

5 ounces frozen chopped spinach, thawed and squeezed dry

4 eggs

6 egg whites

2 teaspoons water

1 tablespoon chopped fresh thyme

1 tablespoon chopped fresh oregano or marjoram

½ teaspoon salt

    Pinch of ground black pepper

Coat a large ovenproof nonstick skillet with cooking spray. Warm over medium heat until hot. Add the onions and mushrooms. Sauté for 4 minutes, or until the mushrooms begin to release their liquid.

Add the spinach to the skillet and cook, stirring frequently, for 5 minutes, or until most of the liquid has evaporated.

Meanwhile, in a medium bowl, beat together the eggs, egg whites, water, thyme, oregano or marjoram, salt, and pepper. Add to the skillet and swirl to evenly distribute the mixture. Cook over medium heat for 5 minutes, gently lifting the egg mixture from the sides of the skillet with a spatula as it becomes set. Cook until the eggs are set on the bottom but still moist on the top. Remove from the heat.

Wrap the handle of the skillet with 2 layers of heavy foil. Broil 4" from the heat for 1 minute, or until the top is golden.

Use a spatula to loosen the frittata from the skillet and slide it onto a serving plate. Cut into wedges and serve.

Makes 4 servings

Per serving: 123 calories, 5.2 g total fat (39% of calories), 13.1 g protein, 5.7 g carbohydrates, 0.7 g dietary fiber, 213 mg cholesterol, 434 mg sodium

Stuffed Spaghetti Squash

2 small spaghetti squash, halved lengthwise

1 tablespoon olive oil

1 large red bell pepper, chopped

1 cup fresh or frozen peas

½ cup chopped scallions

2 cloves garlic, minced

1 teaspoon dried oregano

1 teaspoon dried mint

1½ cups tomato juice

1 cup couscous

4 ounces crumbled feta cheese

Place the squash cut side down on a microwaveable plate. Microwave on high power for 10 to 12 minutes, or until the squash is easily pierced with a fork. Allow to cool and discard the seeds. With a fork, separate the flesh into strands and place in a large bowl. Reserve the shells.

Preheat the oven to 350°.

In a large nonstick skillet over medium heat, warm the oil. Add the peppers, peas, scallions, garlic, oregano, and mint. Sauté for 5 minutes, or until the vegetables are tender.

Stir in the tomato juice and bring to a boil. Stir in the couscous. Cover, remove from the heat and let stand for 5 minutes, or until the couscous is soft. Fluff with a fork.

Add the couscous mixture and the feta to the squash. Toss to mix well. Divide between the reserved squash shells. Cover each shell with foil, place in a 9" × 13" nonstick baking dish, and bake for 15 to 20 minutes.

Makes 4 servings

Per serving: 369 calories, 10.4 g fat (25% of calories), 14.7 g protein, 56.1 g carbohydrates, 11 g dietary fiber, 25 mg cholesterol, 366 mg sodium

Vegetarian Chili

6 carrots, sliced

4 ribs celery, sliced

2 green bell peppers, chopped

1 large onion, chopped

6 cloves garlic, chopped

1 can (28 ounces) tomatoes, finely chopped

1 can (8¾ ounces) corn

1 can (15½ ounces) pinto beans, rinsed and drained

2 tablespoons red wine vinegar

1 tablespoon chili powder

1 teaspoon ground cumin

1 teaspoon ground coriander

5 cups hot cooked brown rice

In an 8-quart pot over medium heat, bring 1 cup water to a simmer. Add the carrots and celery and cook for about 15 minutes.

Add the peppers, onion, garlic, and tomatoes and cook for about 30 minutes.

Add the corn, beans, vinegar, chili powder, cumin, and coriander and cook for about 10 minutes. Serve over the rice.

Makes 7 servings

Per serving: 169 calories, 1 g fat (1% of calories), 6 g protein, 34 g carbohydrates, 9 g dietary fiber, 0 mg cholesterol

Vegetable Strudel

2 tablespoons finely chopped shallots or onions

1 cup sliced shiitake or cremini mushrooms

¼ cup dry sherry or vegetable broth

1½ teaspoons lemon juice

½ teaspoon dried tarragon

1 cup vegetable broth

1 tablespoon cornstarch

Salt and ground black pepper

1 leek (white part only), thinly sliced

1 medium red bell pepper, chopped

2 cloves garlic, minced

1 medium sweet potato, cubed and steamed until tender

1 cup broccoli florets, steamed until crisp-tender

½ cup shredded reduced-fat Swiss cheese

¼ cup grated reduced-fat Parmesan cheese

4 sheets phyllo dough, thawed

1 tablespoon melted margarine (optional)

Fresh tarragon or parsley sprigs

Coat a medium saucepan with cooking spray and warm over medium heat. Add the shallots or onions and the mushrooms. Sauté for 2 minutes. Stir in the sherry or broth, lemon juice, and tarragon. Bring to a boil. Reduce the heat to low, cover, and simmer for 2 minutes. Uncover and cook over medium heat until the mixture is almost dry.

Add ¾ cup of the broth and bring to a boil. Dissolve the cornstarch in the remaining ¼ cup broth and stir into the boiling mixture. Cook and stir for 1 minute, or until thickened. Remove from the heat, set aside and keep warm.

Coat a large nonstick skillet with cooking spray. Warm over medium heat until hot. Add the leeks, red pepper, and garlic. Sauté for 3 to 5 minutes, or until the peppers are tender. Add the sweet potatoes, broccoli, and reserved mushroom sauce. Cook over medium heat for 1 minute, or until hot. Stir in the Swiss and Parmesan. Season to taste with the salt and pepper. Remove from the heat and set aside.

Preheat the oven to 350°. Coat a nonstick baking sheet with cooking spray.

On a clean work surface, lay down 1 sheet of the phyllo with the long end facing you. Coat generously with cooking spray. Top with a second sheet and coat with cooking spray. Repeat with the remaining 2 sheets of phyllo.

Spoon the vegetable filling in a 4" strip along the long end of the prepared phyllo, about 4" from the edge. Fold that edge over the filling and continue to roll up in the same direction until completely rolled. (There is no need to fold up the short ends.) Place seam side down on the prepared baking sheet.

Brush the top of the phyllo with the margarine (if using) or coat generously with cooking spray. Bake for 30 minutes, or until lightly browned and crisp. Remove from the oven and let stand for 5 minutes.

Cut the strudel into 4 equal pieces and arrange on serving plates. Garnish with the tarragon or parsley.

Makes 4 servings

Per serving: 193 calories, 3.7 g fat (17% of calories), 10.6 g protein, 28.2 g carbohydrates, 3.9 g dietary fiber, 10 mg cholesterol, 171 mg sodium

Oven Fries

    1 tablespoon extra-virgin olive oil

    1½ tablespoons chopped fresh thyme or rosemary

    ¼ teaspoon ground black pepper

    3 large baking potatoes

Preheat the oven to 475°.

In a large bowl, combine the oil, thyme or rosemary, and black pepper.

Cut each potato lengthwise to make several ½"-thick wedges. Add to the oil mixture and toss to coat.

Coat a 15" × 10" nonstick jelly-roll pan with cooking spray. Place the potatoes in a single layer on the prepared pan. Bake, turning occasionally, for 15 to 20 minutes, or until the potatoes are lightly browned and tender.

Makes 4 servings

Per serving: 196 calories, 3.6 g fat (16% of calories), 3.5 g protein, 38.6 g carbohydrates, 3.8 g dietary fiber, 0 mg cholesterol, 12 mg sodium

VARIATIONS:

- *Seasoned Oven Fries:* Replace the thyme and black pepper with 1 tablespoon crab-boil seasoning.

- *Southwest Oven Fries:* Replace the thyme and black pepper with 1 teaspoon each ground cumin, chili powder, paprika, and dried oregano. Add ¼ teaspoon ground red pepper.

- *Spicy Oven Fries:* Replace the thyme and black pepper with 1 tablespoon coarse mustard, 1 clove minced garlic, 1 teaspoon dried tarragon, ¼ teaspoon paprika, and ⅛ teaspoon ground red pepper.

Sautéed Spinach and Mushrooms

1 teaspoon olive oil

1 teaspoon toasted sesame oil

1½ cups sliced mushrooms

1 sweet onion, thinly sliced

2 cloves garlic, sliced

1 package (10 ounces) frozen chopped spinach, thawed and squeezed dry

½ teaspoon minced fresh ginger

2 teaspoons reduced-sodium soy sauce

In a medium saucepan over low heat, warm the olive oil and sesame oil. Add the mushrooms, onions, and garlic. Sauté for 15 to 20 minutes, or until the onions and mushrooms are soft.

Add the spinach, ginger, and soy sauce. Cover and cook for 10 minutes, or until the spinach is hot.

Makes 4 servings

Per serving: 67 calories, 2.6 g fat (31% of calories), 3.1 g protein, 9.6 g carbohydrates, 1.4 g dietary fiber, 0 mg cholesterol, 132 mg sodium

Savory Simmered Carrots

5 medium carrots, sliced on the diagonal

¼ cup fat-free beef broth

¼ cup chopped fresh parsley

⅛ teaspoon salt

⅛ teaspoon ground black pepper

Place the carrots in a medium saucepan. Pour in the broth and bring to a boil over high heat. Reduce the heat to medium-low, cover, and simmer, stirring occasionally, for 15 to 20 minutes, or until the carrots are tender. Drain any remaining broth. Sprinkle with the parsley, salt, and pepper.

Makes 4 servings

Per serving: 41 calories, 0.2 g fat (4% of calories), 1.3 g protein, 9.4 g carbohydrates, 2.3 g dietary fiber, 0 mg cholesterol, 104 mg sodium

VARIATIONS:

- *Basil-Garlic Carrots:* Steam the carrots for 5 to 8 minutes, or just until tender. Omit the broth and parsley. In a large nonstick skillet over medium-high heat, warm 1 teaspoon olive oil. Add the carrots, 2 cloves minced garlic, ¼ cup chopped fresh basil, and 1 teaspoon lemon juice. Sauté for 2 to 3 minutes, or until heated through. Sprinkle with ground black pepper.

- *Ginger-Glazed Carrots:* Steam the carrots for 5 to 8 minutes, or just until tender. Omit the broth and parsley. In a medium saucepan, combine ⅔ cup orange juice, 1 teaspoon toasted sesame oil, and 1¼ teaspoons cornstarch. Stir until dissolved. Stirring constantly, add 1 tablespoon honey and bring to a boil over medium heat. Cook and stir for 2 minutes, or until thickened. Stir in ¼ teaspoon ground ginger, a pinch of ground nutmeg, and a pinch of ground cinnamon. Add the carrots and stir to coat.

Spicy Southwest Corn

1 teaspoon olive oil

2 scallions, thinly sliced

½ cup chopped red bell peppers

3 cloves garlic, minced

2 cups fresh or frozen corn

2 cups peeled, seeded, and chopped tomatoes

1 teaspoon chili powder

½ teaspoon ground cumin

½ teaspoon ground coriander

½ teaspoon dried oregano

⅛ teaspoon hot-pepper sauce

In a medium saucepan over medium heat, warm the oil. Add the scallions and red peppers and sauté for 2 minutes.

Stir in the garlic, corn, tomatoes, chili powder, cumin, coriander, oregano, and hot-pepper sauce. Bring to a boil. Reduce the heat to low and cook, stirring occasionally, for 20 minutes, or until the mixture is thickened.

Makes 4 servings

Per serving: 118 calories, 1.8 g fat (12% of calories), 4.2 g protein, 25.7 g carbohydrates, 3.9 g dietary fiber, 0 mg cholesterol, 22 mg sodium

Stuffed Acorn Squash

   3 acorn squash

   ½ cup basmati rice

   Salt

   2 ribs celery, chopped

   ½ shallot, chopped

   1 Granny Smith apple, peeled and chopped

   1 carrot, grated

   ¼ cup pecans, toasted and chopped (see note)

   ½ teaspoon fresh thyme

Preheat the oven to 350°. Coat a baking dish lightly with cooking spray.

Halve the squash and scoop out the seeds. Lay the squash facedown in the prepared baking dish. Bake for about 45 minutes, or until tender.

Meanwhile, in a medium saucepan, cook the rice in 1 cup water and salt to taste. Set aside.

Coat another medium saucepan with cooking spray and cook the celery until translucent. Add the shallot and apple and cook until tender.

Add the cooked vegetables, carrot, pecans, and thyme to the rice and mix well. Keep warm.

Remove the squash from the oven, fill with the rice mixture, and serve.

Makes 6 servings

Per serving: 260 calories, 8 g fat (28% of calories), 5 g protein, 42 g carbohydrates, 8 g fat, 3 g dietary fiber, 0 mg cholesterol

NOTE:

- To toast the nuts, place them in a dry nonstick skillet over medium heat. Toast the nuts, shaking the skillet often, for 3 to 5 minutes, or until fragrant and golden.

Stuffed Tomatoes

½ cup fresh whole wheat bread crumbs

¼ cup grated Parmesan cheese

3 tablespoons chopped fresh basil

1 tablespoon chopped fresh parsley

⅛ teaspoon ground black pepper

2 teaspoons extra-virgin olive oil

3 medium tomatoes

2 cups hot cooked rice

In a small bowl, combine the bread crumbs, Parmesan, basil, parsley, and pepper. Mix well. Add the oil and stir until well-combined.

Slice the tomatoes in half crosswise and squeeze gently to remove the seeds. Place 2 tablespoons of the bread crumb stuffing into each tomato, mounding slightly. Place on a broiler pan or a nonstick baking sheet coated with cooking spray. Broil 4" from the heat for 1 to 2 minutes, or until lightly browned. Serve with the rice.

Makes 6 servings

Per serving: 124 calories, 3.3 g fat (24% of calories), 4 g protein, 19.8 g carbohydrates, 0.9 g dietary fiber, 3 mg cholesterol, 103 mg sodium

NOTES:

- To make fresh bread crumbs, cut bread into cubes and place the cubes in a food processor. Process with on/off turns until crumbs form.
- For a twist of flavor, try fresh lemon, cinnamon, or Thai basil in place of regular basil.

Succotash

2 teaspoons nondiet tub-style margarine or butter

½ cup thinly sliced scallions

1 clove garlic, minced

¾ cup cooked green beans, cut into 1" pieces

½ cup frozen baby lima beans, thawed

½ cup cooked or canned navy beans, rinsed and drained

½ cup fresh or thawed frozen corn

2 teaspoons chopped fresh dill

2 teaspoons chopped fresh parsley

⅛ teaspoon paprika

⅛ teaspoon ground black pepper

In a large nonstick skillet over medium heat, melt the margarine or butter. Add the scallions and sauté for 1 minute.

Stir in the garlic, green beans, lima beans, navy beans, and corn. Sauté over medium heat for 3 minutes, or until the vegetables are cooked and the mixture is hot. Stir in the dill, parsley, paprika, and pepper.

Makes 4 servings

Per serving: 102 calories, 2.2 g fat (18% of calories), 4.8 g protein, 17.4 g carbohydrates, 4 g dietary fiber, 0 mg cholesterol, 35 mg sodium

Twice-Baked Potatoes

4 medium new potatoes

2 tablespoons chopped onions

2 tablespoons finely chopped mushrooms or red bell peppers

¼ teaspoon dried thyme

2 tablespoons buttermilk

2 tablespoons fat-free sour cream

1 tablespoon snipped fresh chives

Pinch of ground black pepper

1 tablespoon shredded reduced-fat sharp Cheddar cheese

Preheat the oven to 375°.

Pierce the potatoes in several places with a fork. Bake the potatoes for about 1 hour, or until they yield to light pressure and are easily pierced with a fork. Set aside to cool.

Meanwhile, coat a small nonstick skillet with cooking spray. Warm the skillet over medium heat until hot. Add the onions, mushrooms or red peppers, and thyme. Sauté for 4 minutes, or until the onions are soft.

Slice ¼" off the top of each potato and scoop out the centers with a spoon, leaving ¼"-thick shells. Place the centers in a medium bowl and mash with a potato masher or fork. Add the onion mixture, buttermilk, sour cream, chives, and black pepper. Stir well.

Spoon the filling into the potato shells and top with the Cheddar. Place the potatoes in an 8" pie plate.

Increase the oven temperature to 475°. Bake the potatoes for 5 minutes, or until the filling is hot and the Cheddar has melted.

Makes 4 servings

Per serving: 234 calories, 0.5 g fat (2% of calories), 5.9 g protein, 52.8 g carbohydrates, 5.2 g dietary fiber, 1 mg cholesterol, 53 mg sodium

Vegetable Terrine

1 large eggplant, peeled and cut into ¼"-thick slices

Salt and freshly ground black pepper

6 cloves garlic, chopped

3 zucchini, cut into ¼"-thick slices

1 large onion, thinly sliced

6 tomatoes, cut into ¼"-thick slices

Chopped fresh basil

Preheat the oven to 350°. Lightly coat a 9" × 11" baking pan with cooking spray.

Place the eggplant in a layer in the bottom of the prepared pan. Season with salt and pepper and the garlic.

Layer the zucchini over the eggplant and season with salt and pepper.

Layer the onion and tomatoes over the zucchini. Sprinkle with the basil.

Repeat the layers until all the ingredients have been used. Cover with aluminum foil and bake for 1 hour, or until the vegetables are tender.

Makes 6 servings

Per serving: 77 calories, 1 g fat (12% of calories), 3 g protein, 14 g carbohydrates, 4 g dietary fiber, 0 mg cholesterol

Mediterranean Green Beans

1 pound green beans, cut into 1" pieces

2 teaspoons butter-flavored sprinkles

2 teaspoons chopped fresh rosemary or basil

1 teaspoon grated lemon rind

1 teaspoon olive oil

⅛ teaspoon ground black pepper

In a large saucepan, bring 1" of water to a boil. Place the beans on a steaming rack and set the rack in the pan. Cover and steam for 5 minutes, or until tender. Place in a large bowl. Sprinkle with the butter-flavored sprinkles, rosemary or basil, lemon rind, oil and pepper. Toss to coat well.

Makes 4 servings

Per serving: 39 calories, 1.3 g fat (30% of calories), 1.4 g protein, 6.5 g carbohydrates, 0.01 g dietary fiber, 0 mg cholesterol, 43 mg sodium

Minted Snap Peas with Peppers

1 teaspoon olive oil

1 red bell pepper, cut into strips

¼ cup chopped fresh mint

1 clove garlic, minced

1 pound snap peas

½ cup fat-free chicken broth

¼ teaspoon ground black pepper

In a medium saucepan over low heat, warm the oil. Add the red peppers, mint, and garlic. Sauté for 3 minutes, or until the peppers are soft.

Stir in the snap peas, broth, and black pepper. Bring to a boil over high heat. Reduce the heat to medium-low, cover, and cook for 4 minutes, or just until the peas are tender.

Makes 4 servings

Per serving: 126 calories, 1.6 g fat (11% of calories), 7.3 g protein, 21.9 g carbohydrates, 1.1 g dietary fiber, 0 mg cholesterol, 46 mg sodium

Applesauce

12 medium apples, peeled, cored, and sliced

1 cup water

½ cup sugar

¼ cup lemon juice (optional)

½ teaspoon ground cinnamon (optional)

¼ teaspoon ground cloves (optional)

⅛ teaspoon ground nutmeg (optional)

In a large stainless steel saucepan, combine the apples, water, and sugar. Stir in the lemon juice, cinnamon, cloves, and nutmeg (if using). Cook over medium heat, occasionally mashing the apples with the back of a wooden spoon, for 20 to 30 minutes, or until the apples are tender and the liquid is reduced. If necessary, drain in a colander lined with cheesecloth.

Cool the applesauce and serve immediately. Or pour into freezer containers, seal, and freeze.

Makes 5 cups

Per ½ cup: 126 calories, 0.5 g fat (3% of calories), 0.2 g protein, 32.8 g carbohydrates, 2.3 g dietary fiber, 0 mg cholesterol, 0.1 mg sodium

NOTES:

- If you leave the applesauce slightly chunky and warm, it makes a wonderful topping for pancakes or waffles.

- For a smoother sauce, put the apples through a food mill.

- This applesauce may be stored in the refrigerator for up to 5 days or in the freezer for up to 6 months.

- To thaw frozen applesauce, place it in the refrigerator until completely thawed. If desired, warm over medium heat or in the microwave.

- To can the applesauce, pour the hot sauce into hot, scalded preserving jars, leaving ½" headspace. Wipe the rims clean, attach the lids, and tightly screw on the caps. Invert the jars for 10 seconds. Store in the refrigerator.

Cherry Compote with Vanilla Custard

Compote

> 4 cups fresh or frozen pitted sour cherries
>
> 5 tablespoons orange juice
>
> 2 tablespoons sugar
>
> ¾ teaspoon ground cinnamon
>
> ¼ teaspoon ground nutmeg
>
> ½ teaspoon grated orange peel

Custard

> 2 tablespoons cornstarch
>
> 2 cups fat-free milk
>
> 2 tablespoons sugar
>
> ¼ cup liquid egg substitute
>
> 2 teaspoons vanilla extract

To make the compote: In a medium saucepan, combine the cherries, orange juice, sugar, cinnamon, nutmeg, and orange peel. Bring to a boil over medium heat. Cover and simmer for 5 minutes. Set aside.

To make the custard: In a small saucepan, dissolve the cornstarch in a small amount of the milk. Whisk in the sugar and remaining milk. Cook over medium heat, stirring constantly, for 5 to 10 minutes, or until the mixture comes to a boil and thickens.

Remove from the heat and whisk in the egg substitute and vanilla. Return to the heat and cook, stirring constantly, for 1 minute. Transfer to a bowl. Serve warm or chilled over the compote.

Makes 6 servings

Per serving: 138 calories, 0.5 g fat (3% of calories), 4.8 g protein, 29.6 g carbohydrates, 1.4 g dietary fiber, 1 mg cholesterol, 63 mg sodium

Melon Sorbet

4 cups frozen cantaloupe, honeydew, or watermelon chunks,
   slightly thawed

1 frozen banana, sliced

1 teaspoon lemon juice

In a food processor or blender, combine the melon, bananas, and
lemon juice. Process until smooth.

Transfer the mixture to a metal or plastic container. Cover and freeze
for 4 hours or overnight. Remove from the freezer and break up the
mixture with a knife. Process briefly in a food processor or blender.
Return to the container, cover, and freeze for at least 30 minutes before serving.

Makes 6 servings

Per serving: 55 calories, 0.4 g fat (6% of calories), 1.1 g protein, 13.5 g carbohydrates, 1.1 g
dietary fiber, 0 mg cholesterol, 10 mg sodium

VARIATIONS:

- *Pineapple Sorbet:* Replace the melon with 4 cups frozen pineapple
  chunks.

- *Mango Sorbet:* Replace the melon with 2¼ cups peeled and coarsely
  chopped fresh or frozen mangoes. Omit the banana and lemon juice.
  Instead, in a food processor or blender, process the mangoes with ½
  cup carbonated water, ⅓ cup honey, and 1 tablespoon lime juice.
  Freeze as directed.

Pineapple Ambrosia

1 container (16 ounces) fat-free vanilla yogurt

1 cup applesauce

1 can (8 ounces) crushed pineapple in juice, well-drained

1 cup blueberries

1 banana, thinly sliced

¼ cup toasted unsweetened coconut

2 tablespoons toasted slivered almonds (see note)

In a large bowl, whisk together the yogurt and applesauce. Fold in the pineapple, blueberries, bananas, coconut, and almonds. Chill for at least 20 minutes.

Makes 6 servings

Per serving: 166 calories, 2.6 g fat (13% of calories), 3.1 g protein, 34.5 g carbohydrates, 2.4 g dietary fiber, 0 mg cholesterol, 39 mg sodium

NOTES:

• If desired, sprinkle with low-fat granola before serving.

• To toast almonds, place them in a dry nonstick skillet over medium heat. Toast the nuts, shaking the skillet often, for 3 to 5 minutes, or until fragrant.

Poached Bananas in Vanilla Sauce

2 cups apple juice

3 tablespoons raisins

1 teaspoon vanilla extract

¾ teaspoon ground cinnamon

⅛ teaspoon ground nutmeg

4 bananas, sliced

¼ cup fat-free vanilla yogurt

In a medium saucepan, combine the apple juice, raisins, vanilla, cinnamon, and nutmeg. Bring to a boil. Reduce the heat to low and simmer for 5 minutes.

Add the bananas, cover, and simmer for 10 minutes, or until the bananas are plump and softened. Remove the pan from the heat. Using a slotted spoon, carefully remove the bananas and divide among 4 dessert bowls. Set aside.

Stir the yogurt into the juice mixture to make a sauce. Spoon over the bananas. Serve warm.

Makes 4 servings

Per serving: 196 calories, 0.8 g fat (3% of calories), 2.3 g protein, 48.4 g carbohydrates, 2.5 g dietary fiber, 0.3 mg cholesterol, 16 mg sodium

Raspberry-Cherry Jam

1½ cups fresh or frozen pitted cherries, pureed

1½ cups fresh or frozen blueberries, pureed

1 cup fresh or frozen raspberries, pureed

⅓ cup apple juice

2 tablespoons lemon juice

⅔ cup sugar

In a food processor or blender, puree the cherries, blueberries, raspberries, apple juice, and lemon juice until smooth. Transfer to a medium stainless steel saucepan and bring to a boil over high heat, stirring frequently. Stir in the sugar and return to a full boil. Cook, stirring occasionally, for 25 minutes, or until the jam is thick and sticky.

Pour into hot, scalded preserving jars, leaving ¼" headspace. Wipe the rims clean, attach the lids, and tightly screw on the caps. Invert the jars for 10 seconds.

Cool on a rack. Store in the refrigerator.

Makes 3 cups

Per tablespoon: 18 calories, 0.05 g fat (2% of calories), 0.1 g protein, 4.6 g carbohydrates, 0.3 g dietary fiber, 0 mg cholesterol, 0.5 mg sodium

Sparkling Fruit Salad with Mint

1 cup sliced peaches

1 cup white seedless grapes

1 cup blueberries

½ cup honeydew melon balls

½ cup small strawberries, hulled

1½ teaspoons chopped fresh mint

¼ cup frozen apple juice concentrate

¼ cup sparkling water or club soda

In a medium bowl, gently toss the peaches, grapes, blueberries, melon balls, strawberries, and mint.

In a measuring cup, combine the frozen juice concentrate and sparkling water or club soda. Pour over the fruit. Serve immediately.

Makes 4 servings

Per serving: 115 calories, 0.6 g fat (4% of calories), 1.1 g protein, 28.8 g carbohydrates, 2.7 g dietary fiber, 0 mg cholesterol, 10 mg sodium

NOTE:

- For a summer picnic, double the recipe and garnish with a few sprigs of fresh mint.

VARIATION:

- *Fresh Fig Salad with Kiwi-Lime Dressing:*Replace the peaches and grapes with 2 cups halved fresh figs. Omit the mint, frozen juice concentrate, and sparkling water. Instead, toss the fruit with 1 tablespoon lime juice. In a food processor or blender, process 1 small peeled and chopped kiwi, 2 tablespoons fat-free mayonnaise, 2 tablespoons fat-free sour cream, 1 tablespoon honey, and 1 tablespoon lime juice. Serve the fruit over torn lettuce; top with the dressing. Sprinkle with chopped pecans.

Angel Food Cake

    1 cup + 2 tablespoons sifted cake flour

  1¼ cups + 2 tablespoons sugar

  12 egg whites, at room temperature

  1¼ teaspoons cream of tartar

   ¼ teaspoon salt

  1½ teaspoons vanilla extract

   ½ teaspoon almond extract

Preheat the oven to 350°.

Sift the flour with ½ cup of the sugar three times. Set aside.

In a clean, dry large bowl, combine the egg whites, cream of tartar, and salt. Using an electric mixer, beat until the egg whites form soft peaks. Gradually beat in the remaining sugar ¼ cup at a time. Add the vanilla and almond extract. Beat until glossy.

Gently fold the flour mixture into the egg-white mixture in 3 stages, folding just enough to mix each time. Gently pour the batter into an ungreased, 9" or 10", straight-sided nonstick tube pan and smooth the surface of the batter evenly.

Bake for 40 to 45 minutes, or until the cake is golden brown. Invert the pan over the top of a heavy long-necked bottle or funnel and let cool for 1½ to 2 hours. Gently remove to a serving platter.

Makes 12 servings

Per serving: 146 calories, 0.1 g fat (1% of calories), 4.4 g protein, 31.7 g carbohydrates, 0.2 g dietary fiber, 0 mg cholesterol, 100 mg sodium

Apple Crisp

Filling

8 cups peeled, cored, and thinly sliced Granny Smith apples

2 tablespoons water

3 tablespoons sugar

½ teaspoon ground cinnamon

Topping

¾ cup rolled oats

½ cup all-purpose flour

⅓ cup packed brown sugar

¾ teaspoon ground cinnamon

1 tablespoon dark corn syrup

1 tablespoon canola oil

2 teaspoons nondiet tub-style margarine or butter, softened

To make the filling: Place the apples and water in a 2-quart baking dish.

In a cup, stir together the sugar and cinnamon. Sprinkle over the apples and toss to coat well.

To make the topping: Preheat the oven to 375°.

In a medium bowl, stir together the oats, flour, brown sugar, and cinnamon. Add the corn syrup, oil, and margarine or butter. Using a fork or pastry blender, mix until crumbly. Sprinkle evenly over the apples.

Bake for 35 to 40 minutes, or until the apples are tender and the topping begins to brown.

Makes 6 servings

Per serving: 276 calories, 4.8 g fat (15% of calories), 3 g protein, 58.2 g carbohydrates, 4.4 g dietary fiber, 0 mg cholesterol, 25 mg sodium

Cherry Clafouti

2½ cups pitted tart red cherries

2 eggs

½ cup liquid egg substitute

⅔ cup fat-free milk

¼ cup honey

½ cup unbleached flour

1 tablespoon canola oil

½ teaspoon vanilla extract

Pinch of salt

Preheat the oven to 400°. Coat a 9" nonstick pie pan with cooking spray. Add the cherries and set aside.

In a food processor or blender, process the eggs, egg substitute, milk, honey, flour, oil, vanilla, and salt until smooth. Stop the machine occasionally to scrape down the sides of the container. Pour the egg mixture over the cherries.

Bake for 25 to 30 minutes, or until puffy and golden.

Makes 6 servings

Per serving: 178 calories, 4.3 g fat (21% of calories), 6.4 g protein, 29.1 g carbohydrates, 1.1 g dietary fiber, 71 mg cholesterol, 72 mg sodium

NOTE:

• For an elegant finish, dust the baked clafouti with confectioners' sugar.

VARIATIONS:

• *Blueberry Clafouti:*Replace the cherries with 2½ cups fresh or frozen blueberries.

• *Apricot-Orange Clafouti:*Replace the cherries with 2½ cups pitted and sliced apricots. Place the apricots in a large bowl with 1 tablespoon orange juice and 1 teaspoon grated orange peel. Soak for 20 to 30 minutes, stirring occasionally. Drain. Place the drained apricots in the pie pan and proceed with the recipe.

Easy Fudge Brownies

1½ cups sugar

⅓ cup nondiet tub-style margarine or butter

¼ cup buttermilk

¾ cup unsweetened Dutch processed or European-style cocoa

2 eggs

2 teaspoons vanilla extract

1¼ cups all-purpose flour

¼ teaspoon baking soda

Preheat the oven to 350°. Coat a 9" × 13" nonstick baking dish with cooking spray and set aside.

In a medium saucepan, combine the sugar, margarine or butter, and buttermilk. Cook and stir over medium heat, bringing the mixture just to the boiling point. Remove from the heat. Stir in the cocoa until the mixture is smooth.

Stir in the eggs one at a time. Stir in the vanilla. Add the flour and baking soda. Mix just until combined.

Spoon the batter into the prepared baking dish. Bake for 18 to 20 minutes, or until the brownies are set and still seem slightly sticky. Remove from the oven and cool in the pan before cutting.

Makes 24

Per brownie: 108 calories, 3.3 g fat (26% of calories), 1.8 g protein, 19.3 g carbohydrates, 0.2 g dietary fiber, 18 mg cholesterol, 57 mg sodium

VARIATIONS:

- *Easy Fudge-Nut Brownies:*Add ½ cup finely chopped toasted walnuts or pecans to the batter.
- *Peanut Butter or Chocolate Chip Brownies:*Add ½ cup semisweet peanut butter or white chocolate chips to the batter.

Chocolate Crêpes with Raspberry Sauce

Sauce

> 1 package (10 ounces) frozen unsweetened raspberries (about 1½ cups)
>
> 6 tablespoons sugar or honey

Crêpes

> ½ cup all-purpose flour
>
> 2 tablespoons unsweetened cocoa powder, sifted
>
> 1½ tablespoons sugar
>
> 1¼ cups fat-free milk
>
> 1½ teaspoons canola oil
>
> 1 egg
>
> 2 egg whites
>
> 1 pint fat-free chocolate or vanilla frozen yogurt
>
> ½ cup fresh raspberries (optional)

To make the sauce: Place the raspberries and sugar or honey in a medium saucepan. Cook over medium heat for 5 minutes, or until the berries release their juice and are no longer frozen.

Transfer to a food processor or blender and process until smooth. Press the mixture through a strainer or fine sieve. Remove and discard the seeds. (This should yield about ¾ cup sauce.)

To make the crêpes: In a medium bowl, combine the flour, cocoa, and sugar.

In another medium bowl, whisk together the milk, oil, egg, and egg whites. Whisk the milk mixture into the flour mixture, mixing until well-blended. Cover and refrigerate the batter for 1 hour.

Coat an 8" nonstick, slope-sided nonstick skillet with cooking spray. Warm the skillet over medium heat until hot. Pour in ¼ cup of the batter, quickly tilting the pan in all directions to evenly spread the batter into a circle. Cook the crêpe for about 1 minute, or until the bottom is lightly golden. Carefully flip the crêpe over and cook for 1 minute longer.

Transfer the cooked crêpe to a piece of wax paper. Repeat the process until all the batter is used, stacking each crêpe between pieces of wax paper.

To assemble, spoon ¼ cup of the frozen yogurt evenly down the center of each crêpe. Fold over one side, then the other. Place the crêpes, seam side down, on a freezer-safe plate. Freeze for 10 minutes. Serve with the raspberry sauce and raspberries (if using).

Makes 4 servings

Per serving (2 crêpes): 346 calories, 3.9 g fat (10% of calories), 12.8 g protein, 67.9 g carbohydrates, 4.3 g dietary fiber, 54 mg cholesterol, 145 mg sodium

NOTES:

- To freeze any leftover crêpes, stack them between sheets of wax paper and tightly wrap in plastic.

- A crêpe pan works best for cooking crêpes. If you don't have one, a slope-sided skillet works fine (most nonstick skillets are slope-sided). Avoid using a skillet with straight sides, because it will make it difficult to flip the crêpes without damaging them.

VARIATION:

- *Chocolate Crêpes with Strawberry or Cherry Sauce:* Replace the raspberries with 1 package (12 ounces) frozen unsweetened strawberries or cherries.

Chocolate-Raspberry Roll

Filling

- 1⅓ cups fat-free ricotta cheese
- 2 tablespoons unsweetened Dutch processed or European-style cocoa
- 3 tablespoons confectioners' sugar
- 2 tablespoons raspberry all-fruit spread

Cake Roll

- ½ cup cake flour
- 2 tablespoons unsweetened Dutch processed or European-style cocoa
- ½ teaspoon instant espresso coffee powder
- 2 egg yolks
- ⅓ cup sugar
- 1 teaspoon vanilla extract
- ¼ cup buttermilk
- 3 egg whites
- ½ teaspoon cream of tartar
- ⅓ cup sugar
- Confectioners' sugar (optional)
- 1 cup fresh raspberries (optional)

To make the filling: In a food processor or blender, combine the ricotta, cocoa, confectioners' sugar, and raspberry all-fruit spread. Process until smooth. Set aside.

To make the cake roll: Preheat the oven to 375°. Coat a 15" × 10" non-stick jelly-roll pan with cooking spray. Line the pan with cooking parchment or wax paper. Coat the paper with cooking spray and set aside.

In a small bowl, sift together the flour, cocoa, and coffee powder.

In a medium bowl, using an electric mixer or a whisk, beat the egg yolks and sugar until light and lemon colored. Beat in the vanilla and buttermilk. Beat the flour mixture into the egg mixture until well-blended; set aside.

In a large bowl, combine the egg whites and cream of tartar. Using an electric mixer with clean dry beaters, beat the mixture until soft peaks form. Gradually beat in the sugar.

Fold a third of the egg-white mixture into the batter. Add the remaining egg-white mixture all at once, folding quickly until the mixture is well-blended.

Spoon the batter evenly into the prepared pan. Bake for 12 to 15 minutes, or until the cake springs back when lightly touched.

Remove the cake from the oven and loosen from the sides of the pan with a knife. Invert the pan onto a clean kitchen towel (preferably not terrycloth). Remove the parchment or wax paper. Using a sharp knife, trim the edges of the cake if they are not even. Starting from the short end, roll up the towel and the cake together, jelly-roll style. Transfer the cake to a rack and cool completely.

Gently unroll the cooled cake. Spread the filling evenly over the cake to within ½" of the edges. Then reroll the cake without the towel. Transfer to a serving plate. Refrigerate for at least 30 minutes and up to 1 hour before serving. Dust the cake roll with the confectioners' sugar (if using). Garnish with the raspberries (if using).

Makes 8 servings

Per serving: 173 calories, 1.7 g fat (8% of calories), 8.8 g protein, 33.4 g carbohydrates, 0.2 g dietary fiber, 53 mg cholesterol, 53 mg sodium

VARIATION:

- *Chocolate-Strawberry Roll:*Replace the raspberry all-fruit spread with strawberry all-fruit spread in the filling. Garnish with fresh strawberries.

Fresh Blueberry Pie

2⅓ cup unbleached flour

3 teaspoons baking powder

⅓ cup canola oil

½ cup fat-free milk

1 cup sugar

½ teaspoon grated lemon peel

½ teaspoon cinnamon

4 cups fresh blueberries

Preheat the oven to 425°. Coat a 9" nonstick pie pan with cooking spray and set aside.

In a medium bowl, whisk 2 cups of the flour with the baking powder. Alternately add the oil and milk, stirring until the dough forms a ball.

Divide the dough in half. Place one half on a large piece of wax paper and top with another large piece. Roll out to a 12" circle. Remove the top sheet of paper and gently invert the dough into the prepared pan. Remove the remaining wax paper. Firmly press the dough against the bottom and sides of the pan. Trim the dough that extends over the pan. Add the trimmed pieces to the remaining dough. Roll the dough out to a 12" circle between the wax paper; set aside.

In a large bowl, gently mix the sugar, lemon peel, cinnamon, blueberries, and the remaining ⅓ cup flour. Pour the filling into the pie shell. Remove the top sheet of wax paper and carefully invert the top crust over the pie filling. Fold the edges under. Seal and crimp to form a rim. Using a sharp knife, make slits in the top.

To prevent overbrowning, cover the edge of the crust with a 1½"-wide strip of foil. Bake for 20 minutes. Remove the foil and bake for 15 to 20 minutes, or until golden brown and bubbly. Cool slightly before serving.

Makes 8 servings

Per serving: 357 calories, 9.7 g fat (24% of calories), 4.8 g protein, 64.3 g carbohydrates, 2.9 g dietary fiber, 0.2 mg cholesterol, 137 mg sodium

Lemon Pound Cake

2¼ cups cake flour

1¼ cups sugar

2 teaspoons baking powder

¼ teaspoon baking soda

¼ teaspoon salt

½ cup butter, at room temperature

1 cup fat-free sour cream

¼ cup fat-free milk

2 egg whites

1 teaspoon grated lemon peel

1 teaspoon lemon extract

1 teaspoon vanilla extract

Preheat the oven to 350°. Coat a 9" × 5" nonstick loaf pan with cooking spray and dust lightly with flour.

In a large bowl, combine the flour, sugar, baking powder, baking soda, salt, butter, sour cream, milk, egg whites, lemon peel, lemon extract, and vanilla. Using an electric mixer, mix at low speed for 1 minute, scraping the sides of the bowl often. Mix at medium speed for 2 minutes longer, or until the batter is light and fluffy.

Spoon the batter into the prepared pan and smooth it evenly. Bake for 55 to 65 minutes, or until a wooden pick inserted in the center comes out clean. Cool in the pan for 10 minutes. Turn out onto a rack and cool completely.

Makes 16 servings

Per serving: 186 calories, 5.9 g fat (28% of calories), 2.9 g protein, 30.4 g carbohydrates, 0.4 g dietary fiber, 16 mg cholesterol, 98 mg sodium

Oatmeal-Raisin Cookies

1 cup unbleached flour

½ teaspoon baking soda

1½ cups rolled oats

½ teaspoon ground cinnamon

⅔ cup packed brown sugar

6 tablespoons nondiet tub-style margarine or butter, softened

2 egg whites, lightly beaten

½ cup fat-free milk

1 teaspoon vanilla extract

1 cup raisins

Preheat the oven to 375°. Coat nonstick baking sheets with cooking spray or line with parchment paper and set aside.

Over a medium bowl, sift together the flour and baking soda. Stir in the oats and cinnamon and set aside.

In a large bowl, cream together the brown sugar and margarine or butter. Stir in the egg whites, milk, and vanilla. Gradually add the flour mixture, stirring well after each addition. Fold in the raisins.

Drop by teaspoonfuls onto the prepared baking sheets, leaving 2" between cookies.

Bake for 10 to 12 minutes. Cool on the sheets for 2 minutes. Remove to racks to cool completely.

Makes 40

Per cookie: 65 calories, 2 g fat (26% of calories), 1.2 g protein, 11.1 g carbohydrates, 0.5 g dietary fiber, 0.05 mg cholesterol, 45 mg sodium

Chocolate Ring Cake

2⅓ cups all-purpose flour

⅔ cup unsweetened Dutch processed or European-style cocoa

2 ounces semisweet chocolate, finely grated

2 teaspoons baking powder

¾ teaspoon baking soda

1½ cups sugar

⅔ cup fat-free sour cream

¾ cup liquid egg substitute

2 teaspoons vanilla extract

1 cup fat-free milk

Confectioners' sugar (optional)

Preheat the oven to 350°. Coat a 12-cup nonstick bundt or tube pan with cooking spray and lightly dust the inside with flour. Set aside.

In a small bowl, combine the flour, cocoa, chocolate, baking powder, and baking soda; set aside.

In a medium bowl, beat together the sugar and sour cream for about 2 minutes, or until smooth. Beat in the egg substitute and vanilla. Alternately beat in ½ cup of the milk and half of the flour mixture, ending with the flour mixture. Beat until a smooth batter forms.

Spoon the batter into the prepared pan. Bake for 40 to 45 minutes, or until a wooden pick inserted in the center comes out clean.

Cool in the pan on a rack for 10 minutes. Invert on the rack and remove the pan. Cool completely. Dust with the confectioners' sugar (if using).

Makes 16 servings

Per serving: 181 calories, 1.7 g fat (8% of calories), 5 g protein, 39 g carbohydrates, 0.7 g dietary fiber, 1 mg cholesterol, 137 mg sodium

Herbed Ricotta Cherry Tomatoes

32 cherry tomatoes, stems removed

Salt

10 dry-pack sun-dried tomato halves

¾ cup reduced-fat ricotta cheese

1 tablespoon grated Parmesan cheese

1 tablespoon snipped chives

2 cloves garlic, minced

Pinch of ground black pepper

2 tablespoons finely chopped fresh basil

Cut a thin slice from the top of each cherry tomato. Carefully scoop out the seeds and flesh, leaving the shell intact. Lightly salt the insides of the tomatoes to draw out excess liquid. Invert on a rack to drain for 10 minutes. Rinse the tomatoes and set aside.

Meanwhile, place the sun-dried tomatoes in a small bowl. Cover with boiling water and set aside for 15 minutes, or until softened. Remove the tomatoes from the water. Finely chop them and transfer to a medium bowl. Stir in the ricotta, Parmesan, chives, garlic, and pepper. Mix well.

Spoon the cheese mixture into a pastry bag fitted with a small star tip and pipe the mixture into each cherry tomato. Sprinkle each with a small amount of the basil. Serve chilled or at room temperature.

Makes 8 servings

Per serving (4 tomatoes): 86 calories, 2.5 g fat (24% of calories), 5.1 g protein, 13.1 g carbohydrates, 2.1 g dietary fiber, 8 mg cholesterol, 65 mg sodium

NOTE:

- The sun-dried tomato soaking liquid may be reserved to use in sauces, soups, or other dishes in which a rich tomato flavor is desired. Freeze the liquid in an airtight container until ready to use.

Hummus

1 can (16 ounces) chickpeas, rinsed and drained

⅓ cup nonfat yogurt

¼ cup minced scallions

¼ cup packed finely minced fresh parsley

Juice of 2 lemons

5 teaspoons tahini (see note)

1 tablespoon extra-virgin olive oil

3 cloves garlic, minced

⅛ teaspoon ground black pepper

Dash of reduced-sodium soy sauce

Pinch of ground red pepper

In a food processor or blender, process the chickpeas until smooth. Occasionally stop to scrape down the sides of the bowl if necessary.

Add the yogurt, scallions, parsley, lemon juice, tahini, oil, garlic, black pepper, and soy sauce. Process until smooth and creamy. (If necessary, add a small amount of water or canned bean liquid to achieve the desired consistency.)

Transfer to a serving bowl. Sprinkle with the red pepper. Serve at room temperature.

Makes about 1¾ cups

Per 2 tablespoons: 54 calories, 2.4 g fat (39% of calories), 2.1 g protein, 6.5 g carbohydrates, 0.02 g dietary fiber, 0.1 mg cholesterol, 126 mg sodium

NOTE:
- Tahini, or sesame butter, is available in most supermarkets or Middle Eastern grocery stores.
- Serve this tangy dip with warm wedges of pita bread, whole grain crackers, or crudités.

Zucchini Bites

2 eggs

5 egg whites

4 cups shredded zucchini

1½ cups shredded fat-free mozzarella cheese

1 cup chopped onions

½ cup grated Parmesan cheese

½ cup all-purpose flour

1 tablespoon chopped fresh dill

¼ teaspoon baking powder

Preheat the oven to 350°. Coat a 9" × 13" nonstick baking dish with nonstick spray and set aside.

In a large bowl, beat together the eggs and egg whites. Stir in the zucchini, mozzarella, onions, Parmesan, flour, dill, and baking powder.

Spoon the mixture into the prepared dish. Bake for 30 to 35 minutes, or until a wooden pick inserted into the center comes out clean. Cool in the pan for 5 minutes. Cut into 24 squares. Serve warm or cold.

Makes 8 servings

Per serving (3 squares): 137 calories, 3.3 g fat (22% of calories), 15.6 g protein, 10.9 g carbohydrates, 1.1 g dietary fiber, 58 mg cholesterol, 329 mg sodium

VARIATION:

- *Sun-Dried Tomato Zucchini Bites:* Replace the dill with 1 tablespoon chopped fresh basil. Place 8 dry-pack sun-dried tomato halves in a cup or small bowl. Cover with boiling water and let soak for 15 minutes, or until softened. Finely chop and stir into the zucchini mixture.

Spicy Roasted Chickpeas

2 cups canned chickpeas, rinsed and drained

1½ teaspoons extra-virgin olive oil

½ teaspoon ground cumin

½ teaspoon ground coriander

¼ teaspoon ground red pepper

¼ teaspoon ground black pepper

Preheat the oven to 400°. Coat a nonstick baking sheet with cooking spray and set aside.

In a small bowl, toss the chickpeas with the oil, cumin, coriander, red pepper, and black pepper.

Place the chickpeas in a single layer on the prepared baking sheet. Bake for 30 to 40 minutes, or until crisp and golden.

Makes about 2 cups; 8 servings.

Per serving: 50 calories, 1.6 . fat (29% of calories), 2.0 g protein, 7.1 g carbohydrates, 2.1 g dietary fiber, 0 mg cholesterol, 170 mg sodium

VARIATION:

• *Southwestern Roasted Chickpeas:* Replace the coriander with chili powder.

Meatballs in Sweet-and-Hot Sauce

Meatballs

> 10 ounces lean ground turkey breast
>
> 6 ounces extra-lean ground beef
>
> ¼ cup liquid egg substitute
>
> 1 can (8½ ounces) water chestnuts, drained and chopped
>
> ¼ cup thinly sliced scallions
>
> ¼ cup unseasoned dry bread crumbs
>
> ¼ teaspoon ground black pepper

Sauce

> ¾ cup fat-free, reduced-sodium chicken broth
>
> ⅓ cup ketchup
>
> 2 tablespoons brown sugar
>
> ½ teaspoon ground ginger
>
> 2–3 drops hot-pepper sauce
>
> 2 teaspoons cornstarch
>
> 3 tablespoons seasoned rice vinegar

To make the meatballs: Preheat the oven to 400°. Coat a nonstick baking sheet with cooking spray and set aside.

In a large bowl, combine the turkey, beef, egg substitute, water chestnuts, scallions, bread crumbs, and pepper. Mix well. Form the mixture into thirty 1" balls.

Place the meatballs on the prepared baking sheet. Bake for 15 minutes, or until no longer pink in the center when tested with a sharp knife. Keep warm until ready to serve.

To make the sauce: In a small saucepan, whisk together the broth, ketchup, brown sugar, ginger, and hot-pepper sauce. Dissolve the cornstarch in the rice vinegar and stir into the sauce. Cook over medium heat until the mixture comes to boil. Reduce the heat to low. Cook and stir for 1 minute, or until slightly thickened. Pour over the meatballs and gently toss to coat. Serve with toothpicks.

Makes 30

Per meatball: 38 calories, 0.8 g fat (20% of calories), 3.8 g protein, 3.8 g carbohydrates, 0.3 g dietary fiber, 10 mg cholesterol, 57 mg sodium

Spinach-Cheese Quesadillas

1 small onion, finely chopped

1 cup washed and finely chopped fresh spinach

   Pinch of nutmeg

3 tablespoons shredded reduced-fat Cheddar cheese

3 tablespoons shredded reduced-fat Monterey Jack cheese

½ teaspoon chili powder

   Pinch of ground red pepper (optional)

2 large flour tortillas (12" diameter)

Generously coat a large nonstick skillet with cooking spray and warm over medium heat. Add the onions and sauté for 6 minutes, or until lightly browned. Add the spinach and nutmeg. Cook for 1 to 2 minutes, or until the spinach is just wilted and heated through. Transfer to a medium bowl and set aside.

Meanwhile, in a small bowl, stir together the Cheddar, Monterey Jack, chili powder, and pepper (if using). Set aside.

Return the skillet to medium-low heat and place 1 tortilla in the skillet. Quickly spread half of the cheese mixture over the surface of the tortilla. Spread the spinach mixture evenly over the cheese. Sprinkle with the remaining half of the cheese mixture and top with the second tortilla. Using a spatula, gently press the quesadilla to combine the layers.

Cook for 4 minutes per side, or until lightly browned and the cheese is melted. Cool slightly and cut in to wedges. Serve warm, with your favorite salsa.

Makes 8 servings

Per serving: 49 calories, 1.5 g fat (28% of calories), 2.5 g protein, 6.3 g carbohydrates, 0.4 g dietary fiber, 3 mg cholesterol, 106 mg sodium

APPENDIX C

Three-Week Spark Exercise and Fiber Log

Aerobic

Strength

Flexibility

Fibe**R**

Appendix C

Every time you eat fiber, log in an "FR"
Every time you perform a 10-min. exercise "spark" just log in an "A" "S" or "F"

Date:	Date:	Date:	Date:
Date:	Date:	Date:	Date:
Date:	Date:	Date:	Date:

Date:	Date:	Date:	Weekly Total
			A ____
			S ____
			F ____
			FR ____
Date:	Date:	Date:	
			A ____
			S ____
			F ____
			FR ____
Date:	Date:	Date:	
			A ____
			S ____
			F ____
			FR ____

INDEX

A

Abdominal crunches, 110–12
Abdominal fat, 82
Abdominals
  back extensions and, 112–13
  sit-up test for, 73–75
  strength training for, 110–13
Achievements of life, pride in, 204
Adrenaline, 52
Aerobic fitness, 34, 57
  self-test on, 66–69
  in Spark Study 2000, 25, 33, 59
Aerobics, fitness guidelines and, 16
Aerobic Sparks, 35, 100–102
  in evening, 183
  exercise Spark equation and, 79–81, 122
  Feeling the Spark guidelines for, 100–102
  intensity of, 100–102, 191
  interval-training workout (Super Spark), 183–85
  in morning, 183
  Spark Launchpad Lifestyle Test and, 122–23
  suggestions for, 186
  Three-Week Spark Exercise and Fiber Log, 383–85
  in Week One, 150–52, 154, 208, 210

in Week Two, 162–63, 166, 212–13, 215
in Week Three, 183–86, 217, 219–20, 223
Afterburn, 39, 55–56
Aging
  calorie burning and, 53
  growth hormone and, 30, 37–39
  muscle loss and, 69
Angel food cake, 174–75
Antioxidants, 132, 203
Appetite
  cravings and, 200
  decreased by exercise Sparks, 39–40
  fiber and, 47, 128, 137, 138
  reflecting on, in Week Two, 175–76
  Spark Appetite Satiation Test and, 90–93
  Spark Your Appetite Scale and, 91, 137–38, 176
Apples, 174
Arms
  flexibility training for, 118, 195–96
  strength training for, 106–9, 188–89

B

Back, flexibility training for, 118–20, 193–94, 195–96
Back extensions, 112–13

384

Baked goods, lower-fat alternatives for, 143
Beans, 128, 129, 134
Bicep curls, 106–7, 122
Blood pressure, 40, 60, 82
Blood sugar, 56, 60
Body fat. *See* Fat, body
Body image, 48–49
Body twists, 118–19
Body weight, 58–59. *See also* Weight loss and control
Bone health, 69, 144
Breads, 136
   rich in fiber, 129, 131–32
Breakfast, 47, 130
Broccoli, 145
Butter, 140
Butterfly (stretch), 197
Buttocks, strength training for, 109–10, 192–93

C

Caffeine, 178
Cake, angel food, 174–75
Calcium, 144–45
Calf "lift-ups," 187–88
Calories, 129, 139, 140
   burned by exercise, 41, 55, 57
   burned by muscle vs. fat, 41
   campfire analogy for burning of, 49–50
   counting fiber vs., 52
   exercise intensity and, 55
   stored as fat, 53, 139
Calves
   flexibility training for, 118
   strength training for, 187–88
Canadian Society for Exercise Physiology test, 85
Cancer, 60, 130
Carbohydrates, 60, 140
   afterburn and, 55–56
   complex vs. simple, 44, 131
   as fiber source, 46–47
      glycemic index and, 56–57
      high-fiber, 131–33
      increasing consumption of, 128
      muscles' use of, 50, 52, 53, 55–56, 128
      in Spark Food Plan, 30, 41–46
      Spark Fuel and, 50–51, 52
      in weight loss and control, 31, 41–42
Carbon dioxide, 51
Cardiovascular disease. *See* Heart disease
Cat (stretch), 195–96
Cereals
   lower-fat alternatives, 142
   portion size for, 139
   rich in fiber, 129, 131–32
Chair work (exercises), 109–11
   abdominal crunches, 110–11
   for arms, 108–9
   for legs, 109–10, 122
Cheeses, 145
   part-skim, 144
   portion size for, 139
Chicken
   coating for, 173
   cooking methods for, 140
   ground, 174
Chili, 136
China, rural, diet in, 45
Chocolate, 202–3
Cholesterol, 35, 60, 82, 138
   chocolate and, 203
   fiber and, 135
   HDL, 90
   heart disease and, 26, 59, 89–90
   LDL, 26, 45, 89
   medical research on, 59
   Spark Study 2000 and, 26, 59, 60, 89, 90, 158
   "Spark Your Food IQ" Fiber and Cholesterol Test, 87–89
Cooking methods, 140
Cottage cheese, 140

Couscous, 140
Cravings, 200
Croutons, whole wheat, 173

D

Dairy products, 144–45, 148
  lower-fat alternatives, 142
Dancing, in aerobic Sparks, 151,
  162–63, 208, 210, 223
Deltoids, push-up test for, 69–73
Deprivation, 93
Desserts, 44, 200
  lower-fat alternatives, 143
Diabetes, 60, 82, 130
Diets, 147, 199–200
  high-carbohydrate, 31, 41–46
  high-protein, 42–44
  history of, 125–26
  starvation, 50

E

Eggs, frying, 140
Embers. *See* Week One
Emotional eating, 126–27
Energy bars, 203
Energy level, 35, 115, 200
English muffins, oat bran, 173
Evening Sparks, 183
Exercise, 126. *See also* Spark Exercise
  Plan
  body fat burned during, 54–56
  broken up into shorter segments, 17,
    21, 34, 98, 103
  cholesterol level and, 59
  duration of, 54–55
  food needs and, 41
  growth hormone released during, 30,
    37–39, 52, 183
  intensity of, 21, 55, 103, 184, 191
    (*see also Feeling the Spark*
    guidelines)
  mortality rates and, 58–59
  and relationship with food, 146
  responses to word, 32
  self-test on feelings about, 95–96

Spark-like, medical research on,
  33–34, 37, 38, 40
  unrealistic guidelines for, 16–17
  in weight loss and control, 33–34, 37,
    39–40, 41, 50, 53
Exercise Spark equation, 79–81, 122
Exercise Sparks, 200, 201. *See also*
  Aerobic Sparks; Flexibility Sparks;
  Strength-training Sparks
  afterburn and, 39, 55–56
  appetite decreased by, 39–40
  combinations of, 169–70
  metabolism and, 39–40
  in morning, 183
  shorter or longer than 10 minutes,
    156
  Spark Burn and, 52
  Spark Food Plan and, 129
  10-minute, 171–72
  Three-Week Spark Exercise and
    Fiber Log, 383–85
  in Week One, 29, 150–56, 208, 210
  in Week Two, 29, 162–72, 212–13,
    214–15
  in Week Three, 29, 182–97, 217–18,
    219–20, 222–23
Exercise Your Passion test, 95–96

F

Fat, body, 34, 41, 58–59. *See also*
  Weight loss and control
  burning of, 50–56, 128–29
  calories stored as, 53, 139
  dietary fat converted into, 43, 60
  exercise and, 54–56
  high glycemic foods and, 56
  in history, 125–26
  location of, 82
  purpose of, 81–82
  self-test on, 81–84, 86
Fat-free products, 141
Fat people, mortality rates among,
  58–59
Fats, blood, 60, 82. *See also* Cholesterol;
  Triglycerides

Fats, dietary, 52, 59, 135
 converted into body fat, 43, 60
 in dairy products, 144–45
 fat-free or reduced-fat products and,
  141
 fiber and, 47, 50, 128
 in high-protein diets, 44
 lower-fat alternatives and, 143
 in recipes, cutting back on, 140
 reducing consumption of, 139–44,
  148, 173–75
 SF-SB equation and, 50–51, 53, 135
 splurging and, 200
 sugar partnered with, 141
 in Week Two, 173–75
Fatty acids, 82
Feeling the Spark guidelines
 for aerobic Sparks, 100–102
 for flexibility Sparks, 115–17
 for strength-training Sparks, 103–5
Fiber, 31, 158
 appetite and, 47, 128, 137, 138
 ideas for increasing consumption of,
  134–36
 keeping track of, 129–30
 medical research on, 130
 protein sources of, 133–34
 SF-SB equation and, 50, 52
 in Spark Food Plan, 30, 46–47, 128,
  129–36, 147, 157–58, 159, 172–73,
  177
 "Spark Your Food IQ" Fiber and
  Cholesterol Test, 87–89
 Three-Week Spark Exercise and
  Fiber Log, 383–85
Fire and Beyond. *See* Week Three
Fish and shellfish, 145
 lower-fat alternatives, 142–43
 portion size for, 139
 toppings for, 140
Fitness. *See also* Aerobic fitness
 conventional guidelines for, 15–17,
  114
 metabolic, 34, 59–60
 as predictor of longevity, 58–59

Flexibility, 25, 34
 fitness guidelines and, 16
 self-test on, 76–78
Flexibility Sparks, 35, 114–20
 body twists in, 118–19
 butterfly in, 197
 cat in, 195–96
 exercise Spark equation and, 79–81,
  122
 Feeling the Spark guidelines for,
  115–17
 intensity of, 115–17, 191
 leg lifts in, 118
 more movements for, 193–97
 pelvic rock in, 193–94
 as quiet time, 123
 rag doll in, 194–95
 rock 'n' rolling in, 119–20
 sample of, 117–20
 seize the day moment in, 120
 sit and stretch in, 119
 Three-Week Spark Exercise and
  Fiber Log, 383–85
 warm-up in, 117
 in Week One, 155–56, 208
 in Week Two, 165–66, 167–69, 212,
  215
 in Week Three, 218, 220, 222
Flour, whole wheat, 136
Food. *See also* Spark Food Plan;
  specific foods
 changing relationship with,
  146
 emotional eating and, 126–27
 as fuel, 29–30
 "Spark Your Food IQ" Fiber and
  Cholesterol Test, 87–89
Food Sparks. *See also* Spark Food
  Plan
 in Week One, 157–59, 209, 211
 in Week Two, 172–78, 213–14,
  215–16
 in Week Three, 199–204, 218–19,
  221–22, 223–24
Frozen fruit bars, 202

Fruits, 128
  freezing, 135
  portion size for, 139
  rich in fiber, 129, 132
  in Week One, 157–58, 159
Fudgsicle, 203

G

Glucose tolerance, 60
Gluttony, 44
Glycemic index, 56–57
Grains, 128, 135, 172–73
  lower-fat alternatives, 142
  rich in fiber, 129, 131–32
Greece, ancient, 43
Growth hormone (GH), 30, 37–39, 52
  morning Sparks and, 183
  workout duration and, 38–39

H

Hamstrings, flexibility training for, 118,
  119–20
HDL, 90
Heart attacks, 45, 202
Heart disease, 60, 130
  aerobic fitness and, 66
  cholesterol and, 26, 59, 89–90
  fiber and, 47
  location of body fat and, 82
  in rural China, 45
  Spark Study 2000 and, 26
  triglycerides and, 85
Heart rhythm irregularities, 82
High-protein diets, 42–44
Hip raises, 189–90
Hips, flexibility training for, 118–20,
  189–90
Hunger. *See* Appetite

I

Insulin, 39, 45, 56, 60, 82, 138
Intensity, 21, 55, 103, 184. *See also*
  Feeling the Spark guidelines
  correct, importance of working at, 191
  growth hormone surge and, 184

Interval-training workout (Super Spark),
  183–85
Intra-abdominal fat, 82

J

Joint aches and pains, 35

K

K's Spark passages, 18–20, 22–23, 26,
  28, 36, 48–49, 60–61, 62–64,
  96–97, 99–100, 113–14, 120–21,
  124, 126–27, 136–37, 146, 152–54,
  163–64, 171, 175, 177, 180–81,
  198–99, 204, 205
Kindling. *See* Week Two

L

LDL, 26, 45, 89
Leg lifts, 118
Legs
  flexibility training for, 118–19, 197
  strength training for, 109–10, 187–88,
  189–90, 192–93
Legumes, 128, 129, 134
Lifestyle
  active, 33–34
  Spark Launchpad Lifestyle Test and,
  93–96
Liver function, 55–56, 82
Longevity, fitness as predictor of, 58–59

M

Meat
  cooking methods for, 140
  draining off fat from, 140
  lower-fat alternatives, 142–43
  portion size for, 139
Meat loaf, 174
Medical conditions, self-test on, 85–87
Metabolic fitness, 34, 59–60
Metabolism, 29–30, 51, 146
  afterburn and, 39, 55–56
  starvation diets and, 50
Milk, 144–45, 148
Morning Sparks, 183

Mortality rates, 58–59
  aerobic fitness and, 66
Motivation, 64, 147, 163–64
Muffins, 173
Muscles
  aches and pains of, 35
  calories burned by, 41
  carbohydrates used by, 50, 52, 53,
    55–56, 128
  protein and, 43
Muscular strength and endurance, 33,
    34. See also Strength-training
    Sparks
  age-related loss of, 69
  self-test on, 69–75
  in Spark Study 2000, 25

N

Nibbling way of eating, 93, 137–39, 148
  medical research on, 45
Noradrenaline, 52
Nuts, 129, 134

O

Obesity
  mortality rates and, 58–59
  sugar and, 60
Oils, 140
  lower-fat alternatives, 143
  portion size for, 139
Osteoporosis, 144
Oxygen, 30, 51

P

Pasta, 140, 173
  lower-fat alternatives, 142
  portion size for, 139
  rich in fiber, 129, 131–32
Pasta sauces, 134
Peanut butter, portion size for, 139
Peanuts, 202
Pectorals, push-up test for, 69–73
Pelvic rock, 193–94
Personality, self-test on, 94–95
Phytochemicals, 132

Plateaus, 168
Popcorn, 203
Portion control, 139, 148
Postmenopausal women, 69, 144
Postpartum exercise, 72
Potatoes
  baked, topping for, 144
  mashed, as thickener, 174
Poultry. See also Chicken
  lower-fat alternatives, 142–43
  portion size for, 139
Pretzels, 202
  portion size for, 139
Pride, in real achievements of life, 204
Protein, 140
  in ancient Greece, 43
  high-fiber sources of, 133–34
  high-protein diets and, 42–44
  snob appeal of, 43–44
Push-Up Test, 69–73

R

Rag doll (exercise), 194–95
Recipes, 225–378
Reduced-fat products, 141
Resistance training, 33. See also
    Strength-training Sparks
Rice, 136, 140
  portion size for, 139
  rich in fiber, 129, 131–32
Rock 'n' rolling, 119–20
Rolls, whole grain, 174

S

Salad dressings, 144, 174
  lower-fat alternatives, 143
Salads, 136, 175
Satiation. See Appetite
Sauces, 174
  pasta, 134
  portion size for, 139
Seize the day moment, 120
Self-tests, 62–97
  on aerobic fitness, 66–69
  on appetite satiation, 90–93

Self-tests (cont.)
on body fat, 81–84, 86
exercise Spark equation and, 79–81
on flexibility, 76–78
on foods, 87–89
on lifestyle preferences, 93–96
on medical conditions, 85–87
on muscular strength and endurance, 69–75
retaking, 203
Shellfish. See Fish and shellfish
Sit and stretch, 119
Sit-ups, 122
Sit-Up Test, 73–75
Sleep, 35
Smoothies, 173
Snacks, 137–39, 148, 173
lower-fat alternatives, 143
in nibbling way of eating, 45, 93, 137–39, 148
suggestions for, 202–3
Soft drinks, 173
Soups, 174
Soy products, 145
Spark and My Exercise Personality Test, 94–95
Spark Appetite Satiation Test, 90–93
Spark Burn (SB), 30, 51–52, 129. See also Spark Fuel-Spark Burn equation
Spark Exercise Plan, 30, 98–124. See also Aerobic Sparks; Exercise Sparks; Flexibility Sparks; Strength-training Sparks
benefits of, 34–35, 37–40
exercise Spark equation in, 79–81, 122
medical research and, 33–34, 37, 38, 40
SF-SB equation and, 30, 49–53, 128–29, 183–84
Spark Fitness Walking Test, 66–69
Spark Food Plan, 29–30, 41–47, 60, 125–48
appetite and, 91, 93, 137–38
carbohydrates in, 30, 41–46

cravings and, 200
dairy products in, 144–45, 148
easing into, 147–48
fiber in, 30, 46–47, 128, 129–36, 147, 157–58, 159, 172–73, 177
Maintenance Plan, 201–4
nibbling style of eating in, 93, 137–39, 148
portion control in, 139, 148
protein in, 135
reducing fat consumption in, 139–44, 148, 173–75
SF-SB equation and, 30, 49–53, 87, 128–29, 135, 137, 139, 145, 158
snacks recommended for, 202–3
Three-Week Spark Exercise and Fiber Log, 383–85
water intake in, 145–46, 148, 157–58, 159, 173, 177–78
in Week One, 157–59, 209, 211
in Week Two, 172–78, 213–14, 215–216
in Week Three and beyond, 199–204, 218–19, 221–22, 223–24
Spark Fuel (SF), 30, 50–51
keeping high, 128–29
Spark Fuel-Spark Burn equation, 30, 49–53, 128–29, 145, 168
appetite and, 176
dietary fat and, 139
fiber and, 87, 137, 158
interval training and, 183–84
protein and, 135
Spark Launchpad Lifestyle Test, 93–96, 122–23
Spark Strength Test, 69–75
Push-Up Test, 69–73
Sit-Up Test, 73–75
Spark Stretch Text, 76–78
Spark Study 2000, 23–26, 191, 200
diet in, 56–57
exercise in, 57–58, 59
fat-reducing tips from, 140–44

feedback from participants in, 34, 39, 46, 54, 68, 72, 81, 101, 105, 138, 147, 158, 165, 170, 173, 179, 181–82, 205
profile of participants in, 23–24
results of, 25–26, 33, 54, 57, 59, 60, 69, 72, 75, 78, 84, 85, 87, 89, 90, 93, 122, 148, 182, 205–6
self-tests in, 24–25, 65, 69, 72–73, 75, 78
Spark Waist Measurement Test, 81–84, 86
Spark Your Appetite Scale, 91, 137–38, 176
"Spark Your Food IQ" Fiber and Cholesterol Test, 87–89
Spine, flexibility training for, 118–20, 193–94, 195–96
Splurging, 200
Starvation diets, 50
Strawberries, 135
Strength. *See* Muscular strength and endurance
Strength training, 33
fitness guidelines and, 16
Strength-training Sparks, 35, 69, 102–13, 144, 151
abdominal crunches in, 110–12
additional moves for, 186–93
back extensions in, 112–13
biceps curls in, 106–7
buttocks tightener in, 192–93
calf "lift-ups" in, 187–88
chair work in, 108–11
combinations of, 169
exercise Spark equation and, 79–81, 122
Feeling the Spark guidelines for, 103–5
hip raises in, 189–90
individualization of, 123
intensity of, 103–5, 191
moving to heavier weight in, 105, 106, 123, 191
repetitions in, 105–6

sample of, 105–13
Three-Week Spark Exercise and Fiber Log, 383–85
triceps turn in, 188–89
upper-arm toning in, 106–8
in Week One, 154–55, 210
in Week Two, 163, 164, 166–67, 214
in Week Three, 186–93, 217–18, 220, 223
Stress, stretching and, 115
Stress tests, 62–64
Stretching. *See also* Flexibility Sparks
Spark Stretch Text, 76–78
Sugar, blood, 56, 60
Sugars, 44, 131, 141
obesity and, 60
Super Spark, 183–85
Supplements, 145
Sweets, 44, 50
lower-fat alternatives, 143

T

Thighs
flexibility training for, 118–19, 197
strength training for, 109–10, 189–90, 192–93
Thin people, mortality rates among, 58
Three-Week Spark Exercise and Fiber Log, 383–85
Tomato soup, 135
Triceps, push-up test for, 69–73
Triceps turn, 188–89
Triglycerides, 35, 39
risks associated with, 85
Spark Study 2000 and, 26, 60, 158
Turkey, ground, 174

U

Upper body
flexibility training for, 118, 193–94, 195–96
push-up test for, 69–73
strength training for, 106–9, 112–13, 188–89

V

Vegetable(s), 128, 157, 158, 175
  grilling, 135
  ideas for increasing consumption of,
    134, 135, 136
  rich in fiber, 129, 133
  in Week One, 159
Visceral fat, 82
Vitality, 35

W

Waist, flexibility training for, 118–19
Waist size, 40, 58–59
  Spark Waist Measurement Test,
    81–84, 86
Walking, 57, 151, 163
  in exercise Sparks, 102, 208, 210, 212,
    217
  Spark Fitness Walk Test, 66–69
Warm-up, in flexibility Sparks, 117
Water intake, 145–46, 148
  in Week One, 157–58, 159
  in Week Two, 173, 177–78
Week One (Embers), 29, 149–60,
    208–11
  exercise Sparks in, 29, 150–56, 208,
    210
  food Sparks in, 157–59, 209, 211
Week Two (Kindling), 29, 161–79,
    212–16
  exercise Sparks in, 29, 162–72,
    212–13, 214–15

food Sparks in, 172–78, 213–14,
    215–16
  refreshing hunger scale in,
    175–76
Week Three (The Fire and Beyond), 29,
    180–206, 217–24
  exercise Sparks in, 29, 182–97,
    217–18, 219–20, 222–23
  food Sparks in, 199–204, 218–19,
    221–22, 223–24
Weight-bearing exercises, 144. *See also*
    Strength-training Sparks
Weight loss and control, 35
  carbohydrates and, 41–42
  exercise and, 33–34, 37, 39–40, 41,
    50, 53
  fiber and, 46–47, 129
  medical research on, 33–34, 37, 40,
    46–47, 60
  SF-SB equation and, 30, 49–53
  in Spark Study 2000, 26
  sugar and, 60
Wheat germ, 135
Workouts. *See also* Aerobic Sparks;
    Exercise Sparks; Flexibility Sparks;
    Strength-training Sparks
  dividing into shorter segments, 17,
    21, 34, 98, 103

Y

Yogurt, 144
Yogurt cheese, 140

RECIPE INDEX

A

Appetizers and snacks
Herbed Ricotta Cherry Tomatoes, 374
Hummus, 375
Meatballs in Sweet-and-Hot Sauce, 378–79
Southwestern Roasted Chickpeas, 377
Spicy Roasted Chickpeas, 377
Spinach-Cheese Quesadillas, 380
Zucchini Bites, 376
Apples
Apple Crisp, 363
Applesauce, 355
Apple-Walnut Muffins, 247
Pork Chops with Apple-Raisin Relish, 307
Apricots
Apricot-Orange Clafouti, 364

B

Bananas
Banana Bread, 248
Poached Bananas in Vanilla Sauce, 359
Barley. *See* Grains
Beans
Baked Beans, 286–87
Baked Beans with Peppers, 287

Black-Bean Casserole with Cornbread Topping, 334–35
Bow Ties with Greens and Beans, 263
Chicken-and-Bean Enchilada Casserole, 310–11
Chickpea, Eggplant, and Tomato Casserole, 288–89
Chickpea Burgers, 337
Chili con Carne, 290–91
Chili Mole, 291
Eggplant Chili, 291
Hummus, 375
Lima Bean Gratin, 292
Mediterranean Chili con Carne, 291
Mediterranean Green Beans, 353
Mexican Lentils with Peppers, 293
Rice and Beans, 283
Southwestern Black Beans, 295
Southwestern Roasted Chickpeas, 377
Spicy Roasted Chickpeas, 377
Succotash, 350
Three-Bean Picnic Salad, 243
Turkey-and-Bean Burritos, 322–23
Vegetarian Baked Beans, 287
Vegetarian Chili, 341
Beef
All-American Meat Loaf, 296–97
Asian Pepper Steak, 301
Beef-and-Barley Soup, 226

Beef *(cont.)*
Cheesy Meat Loaf, 297
Chili con Carne, 290–91
Chili Mole, 291
Chili Sauce Meat Loaf, 297
Ham Loaf, 297
Italian Pepper Steak, 301
Meatballs in Sweet-and-Hot Sauce,
378–79
Microwave Sloppy Joes, 298–99
Peppers Stuffed with Beef and
Spanish Rice, 302–3
Pepper Steak, 300–301
Pork-and-Beef Loaf, 297
Skillet Goulash, 304–5
Sweet-and-Sour Pepper Steak, 301
Tofu Meat Loaf, 297
Blueberries
Blueberry Clafouti, 364
Fresh Blueberry Pie, 370
Bran
Bran Muffins, 250
Breads. *See also* Muffins
Banana Bread, 248
Basic Scones, 249
Cinnamon Buns with Coffee Glaze,
252–53
French Toast, 256
Herb Dinner Rolls, 254–55
Milwaukee Pumpernickel Bread,
258–59
Sourdough Bread, 260–61
Sourdough Breadsticks, 261
Sourdough Hard Rolls, 261
Whole Wheat Bread, 257
Broccoli
Broccoli and Red Pepper Stir-Fry,
336
Cavatelli with Broccoli, 264
Chicken Paprikash with Broccoli,
312–13
Cream of Broccoli Soup, 233
Penne with Broccoli and Peppers,
270

Burritos
Turkey-and-Bean Burritos, 322–23

C
Cabbage
Cabbage Soup, 227
Rich and Creamy Coleslaw, 240
Carrots
Basil-Garlic Carrots, 346
Carrot Soup, 228
Ginger-Glazed Carrots, 346
Savory Simmered Carrots, 346
Casseroles
Black-Bean Casserole with
Cornbread Topping, 334–35
Chicken-and-Bean Enchilada
Casserole, 310–11
Chickpea, Eggplant, and Tomato
Casserole, 288–89
Cheese
Cheesy Meat Loaf, 297
Herbed Ricotta Cherry Tomatoes,
374
Lima Bean Gratin, 292
Macaroni and Cheese, 267
Pasta with Creamy Parmesan Sauce,
269
Spinach-Cheese Enchiladas, 338
Spinach-Cheese Quesadillas, 380
Tomato Macaroni and Cheese, 267
Cherries
Cherry Clafouti, 364
Cherry Compote with Vanilla
Custard, 356
Chocolate Crêpes with Cherry Sauce,
367
Raspberry-Cherry Jam, 360
Chicken
Chicken-and-Bean Enchilada
Casserole, 310–11
Chicken Gumbo, 230–31
Chicken Paprikash with Broccoli,
312–13
Chicken Piccata with Rice, 314

Chicken Risotto, 276–77
Chicken Thighs with Onion-
    Cranberry Relish, 307
Chunky Chicken-Vegetable Soup, 229
Classic Chicken Noodle Soup, 229
Cobb Salad with Grilled Chicken,
    237
New American Fried Chicken, 315
Roast Chicken with Winter
    Vegetables, 316–17
Texas-Style Chicken Fajitas, 318–19
Chickpeas. *See* Beans
Chili. *See* Beans
Chocolate. *See* Desserts
Coleslaw
    Rich and Creamy Coleslaw, 240
Corn
    Corn Chowder, 232
    Spicy Southwest Corn, 347
    Succotash, 350

D
Desserts
    Angel Food Cake, 362
    Apple Crisp, 363
    Apricot-Orange Clafouti, 364
    Blueberry Clafouti, 364
    Cherry Clafouti, 364
    Chocolate Chip Brownies, 365
    Chocolate Crêpes with Cherry Sauce,
        367
    Chocolate Crêpes with Raspberry
        Sauce, 366–67
    Chocolate Crêpes with Strawberry
        Sauce, 367
    Chocolate-Raspberry Roll, 368–69
    Chocolate Ring Cake, 373
    Chocolate-Strawberry Roll, 369
    Easy Fudge Brownies, 365
    Easy Fudge-Nut Brownies, 365
    Fresh Blueberry Pie, 370
    Lemon Pound Cake, 371
    Oatmeal-Raisin Cookies, 372
    Peanut Butter Brownies, 365

E
Eggplant
    Chickpea, Eggplant, and Tomato
        Casserole, 288–89
    Eggplant Chili, 291
Enchiladas
    Chicken-and-Bean Enchilada
        Casserole, 310–11
    Spinach-Cheese Enchiladas, 338

F
Fajitas
    Texas-Style Chicken Fajitas, 318–19
Fennel
    Couscous with Tomato, Fennel, and
        Shrimp, 275
Figs
    Fresh Fig Salad with Kiwi-Lime
        Dressing, 361
Fish and shellfish
    Blackened Catfish, 325
    Broiled Sea Scallops with Ginger,
        330
    Couscous with Tomato, Fennel, and
        Shrimp, 275
    Crab Cakes, 329
    Linguine with White Clam Sauce,
        266
    Mediterranean Pasta with Shrimp,
        268
    Orange Roughy Caribbean, 326
    Oven-Blackened Catfish, 325
    Paella, 280–81
    Pasta with Scallops, 268
    Scallop-and-Vegetable Stir-Fry, 333
    Seafood Salad, 245
    Sea-Scallop Scampi, 331
    Shrimp-and-Vegetable Stir-Fry,
        332–33
    Skinny Shrimp Scampi, 331
    Stuffed Flounder, 327
    Tangy Tuna Salad, 245
    Teriyaki Tuna, 328
    Tuna Salad, 245

Frittata
   Spinach-and-Mushroom Frittata, 339
Fruits. *See also specific fruits*
   Sparkling Fruit Salad with Mint, 361

G

Goulash
   Skillet Goulash, 304–5
   Skillet Pork Goulash, 305
Grains
   Beef-and-Barley Soup, 226
   Chicken Piccata with Rice, 314
   Chicken Risotto, 276–77
   Curried Brown Rice with Mushrooms
     and Peas, 278
   Italian Wild Rice Pilaf, 279
   Lamb-and-Barley Soup, 226
   Lamb with Lemon Rice and Mint
     Sauce, 308–9
   Mixed-Grain Stuffed Peppers, 303
   Paella, 280–81
   Peppers Stuffed with Beef and
     Spanish Rice, 302–3
   Pork Fried Rice, 282
   Rice and Beans, 283
   Spanish Rice, 284
   Wild Rice and Mushroom Pilaf, 285

H

Ham
   Ham Loaf, 297
   Split Pea Soup with Ham, 235

J

Jam
   Raspberry-Cherry Jam, 360
Jambalaya
   Turkey and Sausage Jambalaya, 324

L

Lamb
   Lamb-and-Barley Soup, 226
   Lamb with Jalapeño Mint Sauce, 309
   Lamb with Lemon Rice and Mint
     Sauce, 308–9
   Lamb with Mint Chutney, 309
   Mediterranean Chile con Carne,
     291
Lentils. *See* Beans

M

Mangoes
   Mango Sorbet, 357
Meatballs
   Meatballs in Sweet-and-Hot Sauce,
     378–79
   Spaghetti and Meatballs, 272–73
Meat loaf. *See* Beef; Pork
Melons
   Melon Sorbet, 357
Muffins
   Apple-Walnut Muffins, 247
   Bran Muffins, 250
   Corn Muffins, 251
Mushrooms
   Curried Brown Rice with Mushrooms
     and Peas, 278
   Sautéed Spinach and Mushrooms,
     345
   Spinach-and-Mushroom Frittata,
     339
   Wild Rice and Mushroom Pilaf, 285

O

Oranges
   Apricot-Orange Clafouti, 364
   Orange-Braised Pork Tenderloins,
     306
   Spinach and Mandarin Orange Salad,
     242

P

Paella, 280–81
Pasta
   Baked Ziti, 262
   Bow Ties with Greens and Beans,
     263
   Cavatelli with Broccoli, 264
   Classic Chicken Noodle Soup, 229
   Classic Lasagna, 265

Couscous with Tomato, Fennel, and Shrimp, 275
Linguine with White Clam Sauce, 266
Macaroni and Cheese, 267
Macaroni Salad, 239
Mediterranean Pasta with Shrimp, 268
Orzo-Stuffed Peppers, 303
Pasta with Creamy Parmesan Sauce, 269
Pasta with Scallops, 268
Penne with Broccoli and Peppers, 270
Spaghetti and Meatballs, 272–73
Stuffed Shells Florentine, 271
Tomato Macaroni and Cheese, 267
Tricolor Pasta and Spinach Salad, 244
Vegetable Pasta Sauce, 274
Peas
Curried Brown Rice with Mushrooms and Peas, 278
Minted Snap Peas with Peppers, 354
Savory Split Peas, 294
Split Pea Soup, 235
Split Pea Soup with Ham, 235
Peppers
Asian Pepper Steak, 301
Baked Beans with Peppers, 287
Broccoli and Red Pepper Stir-Fry, 336
Italian Pepper Steak, 301
Mexican Lentils with Peppers, 293
Minted Snap Peas with Peppers, 354
Mixed-Grain Stuffed Peppers, 303
Orzo-Stuffed Peppers, 303
Penne with Broccoli and Peppers, 270
Peppers Stuffed with Beef and Spanish Rice, 302–3
Pepper Steak, 300–301
Sweet-and-Sour Pepper Steak, 301
Pineapple
Pineapple Ambrosia, 358
Pineapple Sorbet, 357

Pork
Ham Loaf, 297
Orange-Braised Pork Tenderloins, 306
Pork-and-Beef Loaf, 297
Pork Chops with Apple-Raisin Relish, 307
Pork Fried Rice, 282
Pork Tenderloin with Honey-Mint Sauce, 309
Skillet Pork Goulash, 305
Split Pea Soup with Ham, 235
Potatoes
Oven Fries, 344
Seasoned Oven Fries, 344
Southwest Oven Fries, 344
Spicy Oven Fries, 344
Twice-Baked Potatoes, 351

Q

Quesadillas
Spinach-Cheese Quesadillas, 380

R

Raspberries
Chocolate Crêpes with Raspberry Sauce, 366–67
Chocolate-Raspberry Roll, 368–69
Raspberry-Cherry Jam, 360
Rice. *See* Grains

S

Salads
Cobb Salad with Grilled Chicken, 237
Fresh Fig Salad with Kiwi-Lime Dressing, 361
Karla's Spinach Salad, 238
Macaroni Salad, 239
Rich and Creamy Coleslaw, 240
Roasted-Vegetable Salad, 241
Seafood Salad, 245
Sparkling Fruit Salad with Mint, 361
Spinach and Mandarin Orange Salad, 242

Salads (*cont.*)
  Tangy Tuna Salad, 245
  Three-Bean Picnic Salad, 243
  Tricolor Pasta and Spinach Salad, 244
  Tuna Salad, 245
  Waldorf Salad, 246
Sandwiches
  Barbecued Turkey Sandwiches,
    320–21
  Chickpea Burgers, 337
  Microwave Sloppy Joes, 288–89
Sauces
  Chocolate Crêpes with Cherry Sauce,
    367
  Chocolate Crêpes with Raspberry
    Sauce, 366–67
  Chocolate Crêpes with Strawberry
    Sauce, 367
  Lamb with Jalapeño Mint Sauce, 309
  Lamb with Lemon Rice and Mint
    Sauce, 308–9
  Linguine with White Clam Sauce,
    266
  Pasta with Creamy Parmesan Sauce,
    269
  Poached Bananas in Vanilla Sauce,
    359
  Pork Tenderloin with Honey-Mint
    Sauce, 309
  Vegetable Pasta Sauce, 274
Sorbets
  Mango Sorbet, 357
  Melon Sorbet, 357
  Pineapple Sorbet, 357
Soups
  Beef-and-Barley Soup, 226
  Cabbage Soup, 227
  Carrot Soup, 228
  Chicken Gumbo, 230–31
  Chunky Chicken-Vegetable Soup, 229
  Classic Chicken Noodle Soup, 229
  Corn Chowder, 232
  Cream of Broccoli Soup, 233
  Italian Minestrone, 234

  Lamb-and-Barley Soup, 226
  Split Pea Soup, 235
  Split Pea Soup with Ham, 235
  Tomato Soup, 236
Spinach
  Karla's Spinach Salad, 238
  Sautéed Spinach and Mushrooms,
    345
  Spinach and Mandarin Orange Salad,
    242
  Spinach-and-Mushroom Frittata,
    339
  Spinach-Cheese Enchiladas, 338
  Spinach-Cheese Quesadillas, 380
  Stuffed Shells Florentine, 271
  Tricolor Pasta and Spinach Salad,
    244
Squash
  Stuffed Acorn Squash, 348
  Stuffed Spaghetti Squash, 340
Stir-fries
  Broccoli and Red Pepper Stir-Fry,
    336
  Scallop-and-Vegetable Stir-Fry, 333
  Shrimp-and-Vegetable Stir-Fry,
    332–33
Strawberries
  Chocolate Crêpes with Strawberry
    Sauce, 367
  Chocolate-Strawberry Roll, 369

T
Tofu
  Tofu Meat Loaf, 297
Tomatoes
  Chickpea, Eggplant, and Tomato
    Casserole, 288–89
  Couscous with Tomato, Fennel, and
    Shrimp, 275
  Herbed Ricotta Cherry Tomatoes,
    374
  Stuffed Tomatoes, 349
  Tomato Macaroni and Cheese, 267
  Tomato Soup, 236

Turkey
  Barbecued Turkey Sandwiches,
    320–21
  Meatballs in Sweet-and-Hot Sauce,
    378–79
  Spaghetti and Meatballs, 272–73
  Turkey-and-Bean Burritos, 322–23
  Turkey and Sausage Jambalaya, 324

V
Vegetables. *See also specific vegetables*
  Chunky Chicken-Vegetable Soup,
    229

Roast Chicken with Winter
  Vegetables, 316–17
Roasted-Vegetable Salad, 241
Scallop-and-Vegetable Stir-Fry, 333
Shrimp-and-Vegetable Stir-Fry,
  332–33
Vegetable Pasta Sauce, 274
Vegetable Strudel, 342–43
Vegetable Terrine, 352

Z
Zucchini
  Zucchini Bites, 376

Conversion Chart

These equivalents have been slightly rounded to make measuring easier.

VOLUME MEASUREMENTS				WEIGHT MEASUREMENTS			LENGTH MEASUREMENTS	
U.S.	*Imperial*	*Metric*		*U.S.*	*Metric*		*U.S.*	*Metric*
¼ tsp	–	1 ml		1 oz	30 g		¼"	0.6 cm
½ tsp	–	2 ml		2 oz	60 g		½"	1.25 cm
1 tsp	–	5 ml		4 oz (¼ lb)	115 g		1"	2.5 cm
1 Tbsp	–	15 ml		5 oz (⅓ lb)	145 g		2"	5 cm
2 Tbsp (1 oz)	1 fl oz	30 ml		6 oz	170 g		4"	11 cm
¼ cup (2 oz)	2 fl oz	60 ml		7 oz	200 g		6"	15 cm
⅓ cup (3 oz)	3 fl oz	80 ml		8 oz (½ lb)	230 g		8"	20 cm
½ cup (4 oz)	4 fl oz	120 ml		10 oz	285 g		10"	25 cm
⅔ cup (5 oz)	5 fl oz	160 ml		12 oz (¾ lb)	340 g		12" (1')	30 cm
¾ cup (6 oz)	6 fl oz	180 ml		14 oz	400 g			
1 cup (8 oz)	8 fl oz	240 ml		16 oz (1 lb)	455 g			
				2.2 lb	1 kg			

PAN SIZES		TEMPERATURES		
U.S.	*Metric*	*Fahrenheit*	*Centigrade*	*Gas*
8" cake pan	20 × 4 cm sandwich or cake tin	140°	60°	–
9" cake pan	23 × 3.5 cm sandwich or cake tin	160°	70°	–
11" × 7" baking pan	28 × 18 cm baking tin	180°	80°	–
13" × 9" baking pan	32.5 × 23 cm baking tin	225°	105°	¼
15" × 10" baking pan	38 × 25.5 cm baking tin (Swiss roll tin)	250°	120°	½
		275°	135°	1
1½ qt baking dish	1.5 liter baking dish	300°	150°	2
2 qt baking dish	2 liter baking dish	325°	160°	3
2 qt rectangular baking dish	30 × 19 cm baking dish	350°	180°	4
9" pie plate	22 × 4 or 23 × 4 cm pie plate	375°	190°	5
7" or 8" springform pan	18 or 20 cm springform or loose-bottom cake tin	400°	200°	6
		425°	220°	7
9" × 5" loaf pan	23 × 13 cm or 2 lb narrow loaf tin or pâté tin	450°	230°	8
		475°	245°	9
		500°	260°	–